THE SAD SON

CLAIRE B. JOSEPHINE

JOSEPHINE PRESS

Published by Josephine Press, Chicago, Illinois

Cover design by Josephine Press
Stock photos. Posed by models.

Edited by Jennifer Huston of White
Dog Editorial Services
whitedogeditorial.com

ISBN: 978-1-7346998-0-7 (trade paperback)
ISBN: 978-1-7346998-1-4 (e-book)
Library of Congress Control Number: 2020904295

To my eldest son—the most undeniable and multifaceted love of my life.

A NOTE FROM THE AUTHOR

I wrote this book to raise awareness of the many challenges family members face when someone they love is mentally ill. Even though this is a serious topic, I honored my personality and unfiltered tone with a conversational writing style so my story would be entertaining instead of . . . well, just sad. That said, if you're looking for a wholesome, serious, informational book on mental illness, this is not the book for you. However, if you're looking for a raw, humorous (and a little naughty) inside look at what I went through as a mom raising a mentally ill son, then grab a glass of wine and get comfy. And one more thing: if you can't take a joke, set down this book and return under the rock from which you crawled. Consider that last sentence a test.

All places and non-famous names have been changed to protect the innocent and the not-so-innocent.

CLAIRE

1989–1990

*M*y junior year of high school, I failed algebra. Maybe it was because I had a crap teacher. Maybe it was because I stopped doing my homework after my mom promised to pull me from the class but then didn't. Maybe it was because I was a little bitch. Whatever the reason, the entire course of my life changed when I failed algebra in 1989. It was my first and only F.

At my school in Muskogee, Oklahoma, an F meant no sports, and my first failing grade came right before tryouts for the senior cheer and dance squads. This was catastrophic news since my sole purpose in life was epic popularity. I'd been on the cheer or dance team ever since sixth grade. *If I'm not on the cheer team, how will the cute boys at school see my perfect body in bloomers and a miniskirt?* On game days, only the cheerleaders were allowed to wear short skirts to school. Without this discriminatory rule, I'd hardly have a reason to accidentally drop my pencil in the hallway. Hourly. *And if I'm not on the dance team, how will the cute boys see how well I move my hips during half-time performances? Or that I can leap into the air in my skintight leotard and land perfectly in the splits?* Eliminating cheerleader and dancer status would make widespread popularity even more unattainable. I mean, I couldn't get there with my below-average personality unless it was camouflaged by my above-average looks wrapped in a school-approved naughty outfit.

Plus, I knew life was over after high school, so I did what any logical person would do in such a crisis—I switched schools. If I'd stayed, people at my school in Muskogee would've thought I didn't make the team, which would've been one tragedy heaped upon another. So with the help of my parents filling out a simple form, I dodged a humiliating bullet by going to an entirely new school my senior year. It was a stroke of brilliance.

I chose Gunslinger High School in Gunslinger, Oklahoma. Ya can't get any more country than that. Go Broncos. My friend Bridget—who I worked with at the mall —went there, so it seemed like a good idea at the time. Bridget was a supersmart, straitlaced gal; I was neither of those things. I had no idea why a shy, brilliant, Japanese girl wanted to hang out with crazy, stupid me, but she did.

I mouthed off to teachers, occasionally did back handsprings down the halls, and skipped class when I had a hankering for tater tots at Sonic. I plastered the entire interior roof of my car with posters of half-naked men, went pool-hopping in the middle of the night (clothing optional), flashed truck drivers, and may have slightly vandalized someone's house by spray-painting the word *dickhead* across it in five-foot-high letters. That kid really shouldn't have picked on me in science class.

I also knew how to throw a great party without ever inconveniencing my parents. I'd never do that—I loved my parents. Instead, I'd inconvenience *other people's* parents—like

the time I handed ou
house. I mean, her hou
stacks of wood for a b
English. All the party go

The best party I thre
that was for sale. It even
was way easier than I'd a
realtor's open house, jamm
lock when no one was looki
proud to say I cleaned the
animal.

I was also reasonably ____ with money. I supplemented my $3.25 an hour income from my job at a clothing store at the mall by winning questionable dance contests at bars on weekends. Obviously, I had a fake ID—duh. I also got Bridget into bars by telling bouncers ridiculous, fabricated stories about her missing driver's license—stories way too detailed to be untrue. Oh, the good old days.

So even though I was a little twit, I was fun as fuck. Bridget told me life was boring before she met me. Until I came into her life, all she did was study. Like that'll get you anywhere. She scored a thirtysomething on the ACT; I scored an eighteen. Not that I was dumb . . . much. I rocked a solid 2.5 GPA throughout high school, which, incidentally, was the minimum required to participate in sports.

Grades just weren't as critical to me as things like dancing, being popular, and messing around with boys. By the way, those are listed in the exact opposite order of importance to me. I loved boys. And boys, well . . . boys liked making out with me. I had long blonde hair, a great smile, and a perfect body. Even with my impenetrable, Aqua Net–engulfed, Meg Ryan-esque '80s spiral perm I'd say I was

...d my mouth and started spewing ...ow better than to actually say.

...ed me on a temporary basis—basically ... know me. Soon, my foot would set up camp ...th, and they'd realize that I didn't know how to ...basic social norms. Looking back, I honestly don't ...me the kids who didn't like me—which was almost everyone. I don't know what was wrong with me. "If I could turn back time" (I sing in my best Cher voice), I'd slap my younger self. The weird thing is that I'm normal now, if there is such a thing. I reached likability at a sloth-like speed in my twenties. And now that I'm in my forties, I'm a peach. I now wonder why it was so challenging before. It's like I was hit in the head in my twenties and became a different person. You know how you can grow out of an allergy? I grew out of my shit personality. It just took over twenty years.

I was even awkward as a little girl. I was born and spent my early years in Chicago. My childhood best friend was a girl named Rachel, and she was the most popular person to ever walk the face of the earth. She was perfect—big blue eyes, cute little dimples, a petite figure, and a very quick wit. Like if the cast of *Ocean's Eleven* had a baby.

When we were kids, Rachel was cheerleading captain; I was just an average cheerleader. Rachel always had a boyfriend; I never had a boyfriend. Rachel was hilarious; I was comedically challenged. Rachel was a stellar student; I strived for mediocrity. Everybody loved Rachel; nobody really liked me.

But miraculously—astonishingly—Rachel and I were best friends from kindergarten to adulthood. Clearly, I nabbed her before she knew better. We did everything together and had sleepovers every single weekend—until that dreaded day during the summer of 1985 when I moved from Chicago to the time I handed out 500 flyers for a kegger at Bridget's house. I mean, her house was on an acre of land, there were stacks of wood for a bonfire, and her parents didn't speak English. All the party gods had aligned.

The best party I threw back then was at a vacant house that was for sale. It even had a pool! Breaking and entering was way easier than I'd anticipated. I simply attended the realtor's open house, jammed a piece of paper towel in the lock when no one was looking, and ta-da! Hammer time! I'm proud to say I cleaned the house before I left. I'm not an animal.

I was also reasonably responsible with money. I supplemented my $3.25 an hour income from my job at a clothing store at the mall by winning questionable dance contests at bars on weekends. Obviously, I had a fake ID—duh. I also got Bridget into bars by telling bouncers ridiculous, fabricated stories about her missing driver's license—stories way too detailed to be untrue. Oh, the good old days.

So even though I was a little twit, I was fun as fuck. Bridget told me life was boring before she met me. Until I came into her life, all she did was study. Like that'll get you anywhere. She scored a thirtysomething on the ACT; I scored an eighteen. Not that I was dumb . . . much. I rocked a solid 2.5 GPA throughout high school, which, incidentally, was the minimum required to participate in sports.

Grades just weren't as critical to me as things like dancing, being popular, and messing around with boys. By the way, those are listed in the exact opposite order of importance to me. I loved boys. And boys, well . . . boys liked making out with me. I had long blonde hair, a great smile, and a perfect body. Even with my impenetrable, Aqua Net–engulfed, Meg Ryan-esque '80s spiral perm I'd say I was pretty. At least until I opened my mouth and started spewing stuff people think but know better than to actually say.

Popular boys liked me on a temporary basis—basically until they got to know me. Soon, my foot would set up camp in my mouth, and they'd realize that I didn't know how to follow basic social norms. Looking back, I honestly don't blame the kids who didn't like me—which was almost everyone. I don't know what was wrong with me. "If I could turn back time" (I sing in my best Cher voice), I'd slap my younger self. The weird thing is that I'm normal now, if there is such a thing. I reached likability at a sloth-like speed in my twenties. And now that I'm in my forties, I'm a peach. I now wonder why it was so challenging before. It's like I was hit in the head in my twenties and became a different person. You know how you can grow out of an allergy? I grew out of my shit personality. It just took over twenty years.

I was even awkward as a little girl. I was born and spent my early years in Chicago. My childhood best friend was a girl named Rachel, and she was the most popular person to ever walk the face of the earth. She was perfect—big blue eyes, cute little dimples, a petite figure, and a very quick wit. Like if the cast of *Ocean's Eleven* had a baby.

When we were kids, Rachel was cheerleading captain; I was just an average cheerleader. Rachel always had a boyfriend; I never had a boyfriend. Rachel was hilarious; I was comedically challenged. Rachel was a stellar student; I strived for mediocrity. Everybody loved Rachel; nobody really liked me.

But miraculously—astonishingly—Rachel and I were best friends from kindergarten to adulthood. Clearly, I nabbed her before she knew better. We did everything together and had sleepovers every single weekend—until that dreaded day during the summer of 1985 when I moved from Chicago to

Oklahoma after seventh grade. Also known as the worst day ever. After that, Rachel came to Oklahoma a couple times, and I spent summers with her family in Chicago and Lake Geneva, Wisconsin.

Rachel's family had a huge cottage at Lake Geneva. We'd go to the beach, go waterskiing, sneak into bars, and have cookouts. I have so many fond memories of my summers at their cottage. Still to this day, I can't believe how wonderful Rachel's parents were to me. Why did they allow me in their home? And their cottage? For months. Unannounced. That's what dead bolts and peepholes are for.

Even though Rachel and I were extremely close, I was always seeking her approval. I never understood how we were best friends considering my social improprieties. Maybe it was because I've always been, surprisingly, a really good friend. Anyone close to me will attest to that. I'm very loyal, extremely dependable, and would do anything for my friends.

Rachel, on the other hand, loved to torment and play pranks on me. When I'd spend the night at her house, she'd pull various premeditated shenanigans. She loved chasing me through the house with a mannequin head on a stick until I was screaming and cornered in the bathroom. Then she'd pull the bathroom door shut, trapping me in the room where she'd planted a life-sized, realistic-looking witch that she owned for some reason. She'd have the light switch taped down and the doorknob covered in Vaseline. Trapped in the dark, I'd only be able to see the witch's dark figure and bright, glowing eyes, but couldn't escape. Y'know, fun stuff like that.

Rachel also enjoyed making me watch scary movies and telling me that her house was haunted. Then she'd pull out her Ouija board so dead people could pick on me too. She took great pleasure in scaring me. So, yes, occasionally Rachel was a tad mean. Not to anyone else, just me. Like I was her puppy dog—her three-legged, one-eyed mutt. I was just so happy someone as perfect as Rachel would be best friends with someone as mediocre as me. Any torture she bestowed upon me was totally worth it.

Honestly, I owe my wonderful childhood to Rachel. Of all the people I've known in my life, Rachel was the most fun. I wouldn't trade my time with her for anything. We spent so much time together that almost all my happy memories include her. She made life a blast. And no one has ever, or will ever, make me laugh the way Rachel did. No one.

Then, when I was thirteen, my parents dragged me to Oklahoma of all places, and I made new friends. I'm being generous making the word *friend* plural. I never made a friend with a cheerleader or dancer on my team. Every year, they never liked me—not a single one. A cheerleader is supposed to have a filter on her mouth, a smile on her face, and a bow in her hair. I mastered the miniskirt-bloomers thing, but other than that, I didn't fit the cheerleader mold. I was the Tonya Harding of cheerleading.

Still, during my years in cheer and dance, I was popular in the sense that everyone knew who I was—even at a school with over 3,000 students. I stood out in my Chicago clothes in a sea of Laura Ashley dresses. I refused to wear those calf-length monstrosities with lamb print and lace collars. I mean, why would anyone *do that*? I don't know, but they did—they all did. And I never understood. I flaunted my splattered-paint minidresses or acid-washed jeans with a cool blazer and tank top underneath—outfits that screamed, "I am Chicago, hear me roar!" My uncensored clothes matched my uncensored personality. I just never learned how to reel things in Oklahoma–style.

The popular boys liked me in small doses, they just never

wanted me to be their girlfriend. The obnoxious girl was okay to kiss and feel up, as long as there was no follow-through. I never had sex, though. I can count on one hand how many smart moves I made when I was young, and that was one of them. Actually, I can only think of one other thing —taking care of my skin. I guess I only need my thumbs to count the smart things I did back then. Sometimes there were rumors about me having sex, but they weren't true. Where I went to high school, everyone was screwing everyone, but I never let anyone screw me. I'm proud of that. That and my flawless skin.

So I went from a school where everyone knew me to starting my senior year as the new kid . . . on purpose.

During my first week at Gunslinger High School, I immediately connected with a guy named Ben. Ben was insanely adorable with his Patrick Swayze mullet and swagger. He was also a tae kwon do genius. He could do the splits between two chairs, and that was all I needed to know. Everyone loved Ben. He was charismatic, popular, friendly, and had a good head on his shoulders. He was like Tom Cruise before Scientology.

I guess Ben was kinda my first boyfriend if you count an oh maybe, three-week relationship. Then, of course, he got to know me. And, we all know how *that* goes. I could only pretend to be likable for so long. Apparently my record was three weeks. However, Ben did learn one thing about me: I was a really good friend. A week after our relationship ended, I showed up at Ben's house and said, "Listen, I know we're not going to be an item anymore, but I really had fun hanging out with you, soooo, wanna be friends?"

It was like a light switch flipped on, and Ben and I became instant best friends. He called me "Claire Bear," and it felt like we'd been best friends forever. He became my closest friend since Rachel, and we were completely inseparable the whole year. We ate lunch together. We hung out after school together. We partied on the weekends together. We went dancing together. Good Lord, Ben could dance. And when we danced, we danced—filthy, dirty dancing, like our bodies became one. Like we could read each other's mind and sense each other's next move. Which, of course, made us horny as hell and led to the best part of our relationship—the friends with benefits part.

Ben was also a tae kwon do instructor, so he had keys to the local dojo. We would go there after hours and drink and make out like the two horny teenagers that we were. We did everything on that dojo floor, except "it." Ben was an amazing kisser. He was amazing at everything really, but he credits me for his unbelievable skills in the oral sex department. I'll accept that. I was a good teacher. When he'd go down on me, I'd critique his moves like he was a contestant on *Dancing with the Stars.* When we started, he was a six, but by the end of his season, he was a solid ten and earned the Mirrorball trophy. Ben was my oral sex bitch.

When I wasn't with Ben, I was at rock concerts with Bridget. For some reason, Ben didn't share my interest in watching beautiful men sing, so Bridget was my wing woman. Bridget and I saw every major concert imaginable, and every single time, we ended up backstage. Getting backstage was a breeze. I just dressed all sexy and flirted with the guy guarding the entrance. Worked every time. In limited exposure, I was really good with men. During senior year, Bridget and I met KISS, Twisted Sister, Damn Yankees, Bad Company, Slayer, Warrant, Tesla, Poison, Guns N' Roses, and Bonham—just to name a few.

Fun fact number one: I ran into KISS at the mall doing some late-night shopping. We hung out for a bit, and Gene Simmons showed me his tongue.

Fun fact number two: Bad Company and Tommy Shaw

from Styx invited me out, and we partied at a restaurant together.

Fun fact number three: After a concert, the members of Guns N' Roses signed my stomach, and I proudly paraded it at school the next day.

I'm overusing fun facts but they're just so fun!

Fun fact number four: Bridget and I were invited on Tesla's tour bus. Bridget wouldn't go, so I went on it alone, which was really, really stupid. I told you Bridget was smart. When I got on the bus, the guitarist and I started making out. He was so good-looking, but of all the guys I've kissed in my life, he was by far the worst. After a few seconds, I stopped and gave him a puzzled look like, "Is this how rock stars kiss?" He must have decoded my look as "stand up and drop your pants" because that's what he did. I jumped up and hightailed it outta there. Bridget was still standing outside, waiting so innocently and patiently as I ran off the tour bus. I wish I was more like Bridget.

Other than that night, Ben was the only guy I messed around with senior year. I spent so much time with Ben that everyone thought we were an item, but we were really just best buds. Best buds who constantly ripped each other's clothes off, but best buds, nonetheless.

I did, however, have a massive secret crush on an unreachable, way-out-of-my-league boy named Michael McFoxy. He was waaay too hot and popular for an irritating girl like me. Michael and I never talked, but we locked eyes every day as we passed each other in the hallway after fifth period. Michael McFoxy was so beautiful—he looked like young Elvis, but hotter. He had thick, gorgeous, dark brown hair, mesmerizing blue eyes, and a perfect nose—if noses could be perfect. He was also smart. He was that guy who never studied but aced every test. He was very quiet in a mysterious and sexy way. He had the same girlfriend all year, so I never made a move on him. I just told him with my eyes that I wanted him, and when our eyes locked, he never looked away. It was as if his eyes were telling me . . . maybe.

I didn't know it at the time, but failing algebra led to Gunslinger High School, Gunslinger High School led to locking eyes with Michael McFoxy, and locking eyes with Michael McFoxy led to my life changing forever.

As the end of senior year was approaching, I finalized my escape route back to Chicago. Since that dreaded summer day in 1985, when my parents hauled me away from the Windy City, I'd been daydreaming about the moment I could ditch that godforsaken place they call Oklahoma and return to the city I loved—the place where I'd left every fiber of my being behind. I had all my dirty-dancing-contest money saved up, and once high school was over, nothing was going to stop me.

But the week before my return to Chicago, I learned something unexpected—like seriously unexpected. Ben told me he was in love with me. Me. Perfect, adorable, smart, amazing, talented, splits-between-two-chairs Ben was in love with exhausting ME. *Now* he tells me! So what happened? I'll tell you what happened. I left . . . because I was *that* stupid. I moved back to Chicago and said goodbye to the first boy who ever loved me. It's funny that I look back and think that was stupid. We were only seventeen years old for Pete's sake. Seventeen-year-olds don't know what love is. Yet, here I am, in my forties, and I realize that it was real. Obviously, we had a lot of growing up to do, particularly me. However, that entire school year, Ben and I would talk into all hours of the night. We danced perfectly in sync without saying a word. Our sexual chemistry was off the charts. We trusted each other, always wanted to be around each another, and made each other laugh out loud. Our relationship was easy—easy and happy and fun. We just clicked. We had the "it" factor. Since then, of course, I've had great conversations with men. I've danced in sync with men. I've had sexual chemistry with men. I've trusted men. I've laughed with men. I just haven't had all of the above with a man. I miss Ben a lot.

ANNA

1990

*S*o, off to Chi-town I went. I moved the day after high school graduation if that gives you any indication of how much I loved Oklahoma. I moved in with my sister, Alice, who's eleven years older than me. Since she was twenty-four years old when we moved, she never had to suffer through Oklahoma.

Alice lived in an apartment in the heart of the city—right off the Magnificent Mile—where the lights, sounds, and hustle and bustle breathed. The sweet smell of cocoa filled the air from the nearby Blommer chocolate factory. My thoughts were consumed with the order in which I would hit my favorite restaurants. I felt like all my senses were awakened after being dormant for so long.

Alice got the socially awkward seed too, but hers was more extreme, and she never grew out of it. Actually, she planted it, gave it plenty of sunlight, and watered it daily, causing her to become Sovereign Ruler of Earth—goddess of knowledge and wisdom, patroness of all that is correct (dun-dun-dunnn).

Despite our age difference, when I was a little girl, Alice

and I were incredibly close. She was the world's best sister and my favorite person in the universe. She did everything with me. She took me to parks. She French braided my hair. She colored with me. She did puzzles with me. I slept in her room even though I had my own. She was the person who taught me to take care of my skin. She told me not to have sex until after high school. I knew if she said it, it had to be true. She was my Oprah. I miss *that* Alice.

Alice credits herself for me turning out so fabulously. I'll give her some credit since she was wonderful to me when I was little. Alice made sure that I had friends and was always on a cheer or dance team (things she never did), so she assumed I was confident and well liked. I did put up a pretty good facade.

Alice always did sweet things for me when I was growing up. Once she made me a denim bag. In true Alice fashion, she told me that she'd hid a note between the sewn layers of denim, so I couldn't read the note unless the bag was destroyed. She loved to torment me, but it was always in good fun. I thought about that note for over twenty years. I loved that bag, and I loved Alice. And she always let me know she loved me too.

Within a day of my return to Chicago, I pounded the pavement in search of a job. I had been working in retail for two years and loved fashion, so I applied at Bloomingdale's. That pissed off Alice because she thought I was too good for retail. She forced me to go on interviews at law firms—so I did. And I sucked. Ultimately, I got the job I wanted at Bloomingdale's on the Mag Mile in downtown Chicago. I thought that was pretty awesome. Little did I know how much that job would impact my life.

. . .

I was assigned to the Junior's department at Bloomie's. I loved working there from day one. The Junior's department, which was on the main level, was always bustling with people. With multiple TVs hanging on the walls blasting music videos, the ambiance was lively and fun. All these years later, every time I hear C + C Music Factory's "Gonna Make You Sweat (Everybody Dance Now)" my mind still travels back to those days working at Bloomingdale's.

My first day on the job, I was immediately drawn to one of my coworkers. Anna was constantly smiling and giggling and had a radiant aura around her. Even from across the room, I could tell that everyone wanted to be her friend. Coworkers surrounded her, laughed at her jokes, and took an interest in whatever she said. She was like E. F. Hutton wrapped in Jennifer Aniston. She spoke with such confidence and intent, yet she seemed so sincere and sweet. She was tall and lean with snow-white skin, long, wavy, light blonde hair, and defining facial features like full lips and perfect teeth. It was hard for me not to stare at her mouth. Anna was so perfect that I thought she'd never like me. But I was wrong. Anna and I connected instantly, and we did everything together that summer. When we weren't at work, we were at the beach, shopping, or out to eat. Sometimes we went "tiramisu-hopping," going from restaurant to restaurant trying different tiramisus around Chicago. We'd Rollerblade along the lake while eating Ben & Jerry's Chunky Monkey directly from the pint since calories don't count when you're in motion. We'd lay on the beach and talk for hours. She'd talk about her hopes and dreams, I'd talk about the cute boys walking by.

While at work, Anna and I often spent our breaks walking to the nearby 7-Eleven to get Big Gulp-sized Slurpees. It was the best 7-Eleven because they had eight Slurpee flavors that we'd mix all together. Then we'd walk back to Bloomie's, Slurpees in hand, lock ourselves in a dressing room, sit on the floor, and plan our next outing.

Anna was obsessed with sweets. She said it was because her strict Polish parents never allowed her to eat sweets when she was young. She made up for lost time by making her four basic food groups tiramisu, Dove bars, Reese's Peanut Butter Cups, and Slurpees. She never, ever ate vegetables, which she referred to as rabbit food. And she never ate fruit unless it was covered in chocolate. If she ate a meal, it was always a cold sandwich, never hot. Somehow she maintained flawless skin and a fit body despite her horrible eating habits. She was healthy in one respect, though—she worked out daily. She woke up every morning at five to go for a run or to the gym—even if we were out late the night before and she'd only gotten three hours of sleep. She used to say, "I'll sleep when I'm dead."

On the weekends, Anna and I frequented various Chicago bars. Every place we went in Chicago, people seemed to know Anna. Every bar we went to, we'd walk past the hundreds of people waiting in line and the bouncer would give Anna a big hug and kiss, then let us in for free. Everyone seemed to know Anna's name and everyone loved her. We even drank for free because either men would send us drinks or the bartender knew Anna. Free drinks would be a huge score for most, but neither of us were big drinkers.

One might think men loved Anna because she was easy, but nothing was further from the truth. She'd only had sex with one man, a model named William. We'd be out and Anna would see a billboard with his face plastered on it, and she'd be like, "Oh, there's William." His face was everywhere. I met William briefly a couple times when he visited Anna at Bloomingdale's, but he was so consumed with his modeling career that Anna rarely saw him during the year they dated.

Anna's parents couldn't stand William because he wasn't

Polish. They didn't like me either for the same reason. Her parents lived, breathed, and ate only things that were Polish. They spoke only Polish to Anna, so she was fluent. They wouldn't respond to her if she spoke English even though they understood.

Anna graduated from a Catholic high school in a Polish community. Of course, she was Homecoming Queen. One year she was even named queen of the Chicago Polish Parade. If I had to guess, I'd say that was her parents' proudest day.

Anna's parents often voiced their disapproval of her life. Instead of settling down with a nice Polish man making nice Polish babies, Anna wanted to be an actress. Anna had already worked on the movie *Backdraft*, a Pringles commercial, and various other small jobs. She hadn't landed a big role yet, but I knew it was only a matter of time.

Anna wanted to move to California to fully commit her life to acting. Coincidentally, my brother, James, was planning a move from Oklahoma to San Diego at the time. So, James, Anna, and I all moved to San Diego in the fall of 1990, just four months after I'd returned to Chicago.

The three of us enjoyed sharing an apartment, but it didn't take long for Anna to realize that the two-plus-hour drive (without traffic) from San Diego to Los Angeles was unbearable. She had to wake up at three in the morning to work out then drive to Los Angeles to make her morning auditions. So, a few months later, Anna left San Diego and moved to LA. I decided to stay because I was in love! I was in love! I was in love!

DANTE AND DICKS

1990–1991

I fell in love with someone totally and completely not my type. Dante was a comedian. Back in 1990, my brother, James, was taking a stab at stand-up comedy, so I went to all his shows. That's how I met Dante at the Comedy Store in La Jolla. I was there every Tuesday cheering on James for amateur night. Even though Dante was an experienced comedian, he'd try new material on Tuesday nights. Every Tuesday he pursued me, and every Tuesday, I'd turn him down. I just didn't find him attractive, and that was literally my only dating criteria at the time. He had a receding hairline and was kind of short, so what can I say . . . even though my boyfriend history was nonexistent, he wasn't hot enough for a snob like me.

But that damn Dante kept pursuing me and pursuing me and pursuing me. Like a five-foot-nine-inch, bloodsucking parasite—but in a good way. He laid the charm on thick, bringing me flowers in his quest to win my heart. No one had ever, ever pursued me before. But what finally made me cave was that Dante was absolutely hilarious, and I'm a sucker for someone who can make me laugh. So I decided to give Dante a chance, and, ultimately, I fell in love with his great personality. And you know what . . . once I fell in love, I thought he was the hottest guy on the planet.

Dante was a pretty successful comedian who performed with a lot of famous people. Since Dante worked with them, I saw their shows and met them all—except Robin Williams. (Sigh.) Between my brother doing comedy and all of Dante's performances, I was at a comedy show almost every night of the week, and I loved it!

I didn't act or look the part, but I was eighteen and still a virgin. My virginity seemed as believable as Madonna's in her 1984 song. I told Dante I had a six-month no sex rule, meaning that I wouldn't have sex until we were together six months. (My sister suggested that time frame.) My rule didn't deter Dante from dating me, and he treated me like a goddess. He took me to nice restaurants, showered me with gifts, and always made me feel beautiful. He was a complete gentleman and never once pressured me to have sex.

After Dante and I had been dating for about five months, Rachel came to visit me in San Diego, and the three of us had the time of our lives. Put a girl like Rachel and a guy like Dante together, and it was like pairing a fine wine with the perfect cheese. I was the cracker that cleansed the palate of socially acceptable behavior. But at least I was fun. No one ever accused me of being boring. Weird, yes. Annoying, yes. Inappropriate, yes. But never boring.

After six months of Dante wining and dining and spoiling me, we finally did "it." Of course Dante made it special with a candlelit room and a bed covered in rose petals. He was definitely a romantic and made my first time very memorable and sweet. But once we did it, that's all I wanted to do—in every imaginable position and every imaginable location. Once, we even pulled over to the side of the road and did it on the hood of the car in broad daylight. We stayed dressed, of course. Mostly. I mean, I wouldn't want to get dirty.

In the early '90s, that was called living on the edge. This was way before cell phones—can't get away with fun shit like that anymore.

Unfortunately, our sexfest only lasted a month. One glorious month of sex-filled days, Taco Bell–filled afternoons, and comedy-filled nights. But I no longer had a virgin carrot to dangle in front of Dante, and it's not like I had an award-winning personality to keep him hooked. So he dumped me. I was totally and completely shattered.

Two months and fifty pints of Ben & Jerry's later (God I miss my teenage metabolism), I went to visit my parents in Oklahoma. I just wanted to relax, regroup, and move on with my life.

While in Oklahoma, I ran into a guy named Billy, whom I'd worked with briefly during high school. Billy was kinda cute—borderline make-out worthy. He seemed like a really nice guy, the kind of guy you introduce to parents. We enjoyed each other's company and spent a lot of time together during the weeks I was in town.

One night, Billy and I went out with some friends to a dance club. While I hit the dance floor, Billy hung out with the boys. When I was ready to head home, I noticed Billy was acting peculiar. I asked our friends if he'd been drinking, but they said no. I was always exceptionally responsible when it came to drinking and driving, but not exceptionally responsible when it came to trusting my gut. Like an exhausted fool, I jumped into Billy's antique truck and lay down across the giant front seat. Yes, the bastard collected antique trucks. Nice hobby, asshole. You see, antique trucks don't have seatbelts because they're fucking antiques.

Within a few blocks, Billy hit a parked car. My face went flying into the dashboard. I jumped out of the truck and ran back to the dance club covered in blood. I ran into the bathroom and looked at my face in the mirror. *Crap*. My four front teeth were almost completely knocked out—only little stubs were left. And my cute nose—smashed.

A bouncer drove me to a nearby hospital (thank you perfect stranger) where I was told my nose was shattered into a thousand pieces. *That's nice to hear, thank you doctor. Are you sure it's not shattered into a million pieces?*

My parents had just left town on a short business trip for my dad's job, so I called splits-between-two-chairs Ben's parents, and they picked me up at the hospital in the middle of the night and lovingly took care of me for a couple days. No, this is not the part of the story where Ben nurses me back to health and we rekindle our love. Unfortunately, Ben was in a new relationship with a woman, who—spoiler alert —secretly threw away my invitation to their future wedding and wrote "return to sender" on all the Christmas cards I attempted to send him.

While recovering, I decided not to tell Anna about my accident. If she'd found out, she would've dropped everything and flown to Oklahoma to see me. At the time, she was temporarily back in Chicago working on the movie *Batman Returns,* so I didn't want to interrupt her time on the set.

After that awful night, Billy never called me again. He had to scrub my blood off the seats and dashboard of his stupid antique truck. He had to vacuum pieces of my teeth off his floor. But Billy Dix (perfect last name except it's spelled wrong) never checked to see if I was okay. I later found out he was, indeed, drinking that night.

I got veneers on my teeth. I had surgery to reshape my nose. Am I as pretty as before? No, but people are shocked when I tell them my face was bashed into a dashboard. Before the accident, my smile was my best feature. I used to have the biggest smile, like I was the happiest person alive. After the accident, and every day since, I hide my smile. Some of my happiness was permanently ripped away from me that night, along with my confidence—and my ability to eat apples.

I know things could've been worse. They also could've been better. I could've walked away without a scratch like Billy Dicks (that's better) who now flashes his big smile as lead pastor at a church, but has yet to tell me he's sorry. *Praise the Lord!* Meanwhile, I've spent about fifty hours in a dental chair since then, which has cost me tens of thousands of dollars. I've had two sets of veneers and about six root canals, which can lead to various other health problems. Dentists tell me my teeth are slowly dying due to the impact of that accident. I'm dreading the day they fall out completely. It's a recurring nightmare I have. Thanks Pastor Dicks. I hope you enjoyed those drinks.

ANNA AND BATMAN—SUPERHEROES

1991–1993

*I*joined Anna when she returned to Los Angeles. We shared a small apartment with two other people to save on rent. Anna was a crazy workaholic. She would wake up insanely early, go for a run, then go on every audition possible. Audition, after audition, after audition. Then, she'd work as a waitress at night. She never stopped. Never, ever, ever stopped. She was like a superhero whose superpower was boundless energy without healthy food or sleep. To this day, I have never met anyone as driven as Anna.

Since Anna was always busy, I befriended a guy named Devon. I met him at my job waiting tables at the Hollywood Diner. Devon and I often hung out with his friend Angus. Angus, who happened to be the son of world-renowned hairdresser Paul Mitchell, was supercute. Truth be told, I had a bit of a crush on Angus. We had a minifling, but I was back to my standard inability to keep a guy for more than a week. Even though Angus and I weren't an item, the two of us and Devon had a blast together. Like Anna in Chicago, when I was out with Angus we'd hightail it past the hundreds of people in line at the hip nightclubs and get in free. I also got free shampoo, so that was a plus.

One night Angus got us front-row tickets to an INXS concert. Like every woman in the world, I was in love with lead singer Michael Hutchence. After a night of dancing, sitting on Devon's shoulders, and screaming my affections at Michael Hutchence, I decided to do something brilliant. Something totally, utterly brilliant. I jumped up on stage. I mean, I was already in the front row, so he was right there. He was just singing a little ole encore song at the time, so it was no biggie.

Now what I am about to tell you, I swear to Jesus happened. Are you ready? You're not. Sit down. You already are? Of course you are, no one reads standing up. With God as my witness, and like 30,000 other people, Michael Hutchence stopped midsong, grabbed me tight, and started kissing me right there on stage. We full-on made out in the middle of the stage with only background music playing (since you can't sing with your tongue down someone's throat). For five solid minutes. Five miraculous, mind-blowing minutes. I do declare Michael Hutchence is the best kisser to ever walk the face of the earth. Truth.

He slipped a backstage pass into my pocket, and I walked off the side of the stage. Then I got arrested. Well, not officially arrested. Arrested by the wannabe police officers in charge of security at the concert. I was in a dreamy, kissy haze and just remember being brought into a little room for maybe an hour, then they let me go. But by then, it was too late. Michael Hutchence was gone. My love affair with Michael Hutchence lasted only five minutes. That's short—even for me.

. . .

While I was busy living it up with beautiful men, Anna was busy working her ass off. She finally took an evening off work when the day she had been waiting for finally arrived —*Batman Returns* was in theaters. We went to see it opening night in June 1992. Anna worked on that movie for months doing extra work, but she also had a small part as a reporter.

When the movie started, Anna had the biggest smile on her face. As the minutes ticked by, her smile lessened. By the end, she was slouched in her seat. Her reporter scene had been cut. I'd never seen Anna look so disappointed before. For the amount of time she'd spent on that movie, we hardly saw her.

Anna's disappointment didn't set her back for even a minute, though. Her motivation was unwavering. Over the next several months, she continued to work with a lot of big stars, but Sandra Bullock was her favorite. She said Sandra was so genuine and kind. Anna said being like Sandra was her goal—a huge star with a huge heart, who treated everyone with respect. Anna often spoke about all the good she would do with her money if she made it big. She genuinely wanted to make a difference in the world.

Anna only had one sibling, and he was an engineer in Chicago. I'd never met her brother, but Anna spoke very highly of him. He decided to visit Anna briefly when he came to town on a business trip in the fall of '92. They decided to head to Las Vegas for the day. Anna begged me to go, but my boss wouldn't let me off work.

On their drive to Las Vegas, Anna hit a slippery spot in the road and lost control of her car while exiting the expressway. Her car flew off the road and rolled several times down a hill. Thankfully, her brother was resting at the time so his seat was reclined. He was also wearing his seat belt. He walked away from the accident unscathed. Sadly, Anna did not. She, too, was wearing her seat belt, but because her seat was upright when the car rolled, the metal from the roof ripped off her ear and the side of her face was severely slashed.

When I got the news from Anna's brother, my heart sank. I immediately hopped on a flight to Las Vegas and went to the hospital. When I arrived, Anna was resting. It felt sickening to see someone so strong and vivacious sunken into a hospital bed. Her eyes were completely black and blue. She had stitches all the way around her reattached ear and down the side of her face.

I approached quietly then started rubbing Anna's bloody hair. She slowly opened her eyes, looked up at me with her big Anna smile and said, "When are you getting me outta this dump?" I started to laugh and cry then thought to myself, *Only Anna could have an ear ripped off and not complain.*

Immediately upon our return to Los Angeles, Anna still woke up every morning at five to work out (against doctor's orders) and then go on auditions. Even while sporting two black eyes and bloodstained stitches, she continued to compete for roles with hundreds of beautiful women. She never gave up—she was unstoppable. When I told her to rest she said, "resting is for the dead."

MICHAEL

1993

I was twenty-one years old and heading to Chicago to live with friends for the summer of 1993. Even Anna was going to join us because in the '90s, most acting auditions in Los Angeles were on hiatus during the summer months. On my way to Chicago, I stopped in Oklahoma to spend some time with my parents. You'd think by now I'd avoid Oklahoma like the plague, but I didn't.

While visiting, I gave my friend Tammy a call and we made plans to go out. Tammy was the only popular girl at Gunslinger High School who'd given me the time of day senior year. We decided to see a live band at a Muskogee bar.

We arrived at the bar and grabbed a table outside where the band was playing. The sky was full of stars, and the live music was loud enough for a lively atmosphere, but not too loud to have a conversation. While Tammy and I got caught up on what had been going on in each other's lives, I periodically scoped the crowd searching for hot men like any living, breathing, single woman would do.

Suddenly, my eyes stopped. They stopped and widened like Tom spotting Jerry. My mouth began watering. I may have drooled. There, about twenty feet away from me, sat *the* Michael McFoxy. Young Elvis Michael McFoxy. Beautiful, thick, dark hair Michael McFoxy. Mesmerizing, blue eyes Michael McFoxy. Perfect nose Michael McFoxy. Holy shit—it was Michael McFoxy!

I didn't hear another word come out of Tammy's mouth because once I set eyes on Michael McFoxy, everything around me became white noise. He was the unreachable guy I'd locked eyes with every day after fifth period senior year. I'd never had a shot with him during high school, but at this point in my life, I was normal-ish, so I figured that maybe I did. There was only one way to find out.

We—and by *we*, I mean I—decided we no longer wanted our sought-after table and moved to the grassy area closer to Michael McFoxy. *Ah, that's better.* He was just as gorgeous as he was in high school. Even more so, if that was humanly possible.

"Hi!" I said cheerfully when his eyes looked my way. He responded with an unenthusiastic "Hi" and flashed his wedding ring at me. Like, literally, wiggled his ring finger at me. *What the hell?!* Michael McFoxy assumed I wanted him. *What a pompous dick! Perceptive little fucker, but a dick, nonetheless. He got all that from "Hi"? He's been demoted to just Michael.*

Michael and his friend continued their evening, and Tammy and I happily continued ours without the hound dog. After a while, Michael's friend starting talking to us. He was single and probably thought we were pretty.

The four of us ended up talking for a couple hours. Michael seemed to realize that I wasn't quite as annoying as I had been in high school. I assumed this because he changed his story. He said he'd recently gone through a bad divorce and wore his ring so he could go out and women would leave him alone. *Hmm, well, again, what an audacious pig. God forbid women throw themselves at your gorgeousness. But, I'll take it. . . . Michael is no longer married.*

When Michael asked for my number, I gave it to him. But I assumed I would never hear from him again.

Shockingly, Michael called me the next day and asked me out. *Hmm, I thought he wasn't ready for a relationship.* Then I started dancing around the house.

Michael picked me up in a black Jeep Wrangler with the top off, which only made him hotter. He took me to a very fancy restaurant in Muskogee, where I found out he worked. *Well, he must've told me the truth about not being married since he took me to his place of employment for everyone to see. Phew.*

He ordered wine like an aficionado. I found that superhot even though I wasn't a big drinker and knew absolutely nothing about wine. Then he proceeded to order for me, which I found annoying since I took my ordering very seriously. However, I didn't hear what he ordered because I was busy contemplating my level of annoyance.

A fancy mushroom appetizer arrived. *Ick. I hate mushrooms. Crap, now I have to eat mushrooms and pretend I like them. If you were slightly less gorgeous, I could just be honest. Damn your perfect face!*

When our food arrived, I was delighted to see a steak placed in front of me. *Ah, now that's more like it! All is forgiven. I hope it's medium-rare. It is! Good job!*

Our conversation was great, and my meal was delicious. I was starting to think that perhaps I could pull off a date with a stunning man. Actually, I was downright delightful.

Michael drove me back to my house and gave me a very, very nice kiss. *He's hot* and *a great kisser. Uh-oh . . . I'm in trouble.*

Somehow Michael became my boyfriend overnight. We got along extraordinarily well, and, surprisingly, he didn't play games. He called me every day, and we were together every night. He didn't pull the typical hot-guy thing of calling every three days and only going out with me once a week. We were inseparable from our first date on.

Michael always did sweet little things for me, like drop off peanut M&M's or a Slurpee at my house on his way to work. He left cute little notes on my car that said he couldn't wait to see me later. He treated me really well.

Michael was also wicked smart. He devoured books. It seemed like every other day, he was reading a new one. I wasn't much of a reader, so I found that impressive. Michael also spoke intelligently about every imaginable subject, and I hung on his every word. I thought he was brilliant. No wonder he was able to graduate with a bachelor's degree in three years instead of four. By the time he graduated, I hadn't even completed two years of college. But then again, I was earning my degree piece by piece. At that point, I'd already taken classes at three different schools. While I was still figuring things out, Michael was laser-focused. His dream was to become a doctor, so he was applying to medical schools.

Gorgeous. Intelligent. Sweet. Driven. . . . I'd found my perfect man.

I still had my six-month no sex rule, which I was certain would be a game changer for Michael, but (knock me over with a feather) Michael never once pressured me to have sex. He was astonishingly respectful.

About a month into our relationship, Michael told me he loved me, and I'll never forget how he did it. He looked me right in the eyes, told me he loved me with such sincerity, and then put his finger over my mouth to hush me so I wouldn't say it back. Or perhaps he wasn't sure if I would say it back, so he tried to spare himself the rejection. I wasn't sure if I found that sweet, sexy, or sad.

Since I obviously had to stay and see where things went

with Michael, when fall rolled around I got a job waiting tables in Muskogee and enrolled at my fourth college. Hot future doctor trumps Chicago.

During this time, Michael and I were both servers at different restaurants. Every night when he finished work, he would come to my restaurant and wait for my shift to end since I typically worked later than him. Then we usually met up with his friends at a bar, had some drinks, and played pool. Michael was a kickass pool player. *Seriously, is there anything this guy can't do?*

I became more of a partier because I drank a couple beers and smoked a cigarette or two with the guys most nights. I never really smoked before, but Michael and his friends were all social smokers, and I learned I enjoyed a cigarette with my beer. *Who knew?*

A guy named Kevin was one of Michael's best friends. Kevin had been a major dick to me in high school, so it was weird when we started hanging out. We got along all right for Michael's sake, but we secretly hated each other. He had a sweet longtime girlfriend who was way too good for him.

Then there was Michael's friend Paul, who was *so* nice. Paul and I got along perfectly, and I loved him. Paul was the mature father figure in the group. He already owned a nice house and seemed to have his shit together. I felt like Paul liked me a lot—not in a sexual way, but in a I-really-want-to-warn-you-but-can't kind of way. I always felt like he was holding back something that he wanted to tell me. He had a loyalty to Michael that superseded his care for me.

Michael occasionally spoke of his ex-wife, Nicole. He said he'd only married her because she'd gotten pregnant, but then she lost the baby. *Well, it was admirable that he married her when she got pregnant,* I thought. But he said that Nicole was totally psychotic, so he left. Michael told me she threw things at him and hit him. He even had a little scar by his eye that he got when Nicole threw a lamp at his head. Michael was annoyed that he was still paying off Nicole's engagement ring even though they were no longer married. *He buys nice rings. Good to know.*

Michael lived with his father, Michael Sr., and his stepmother, Fannie. I spent the night at their house regularly and got to know Fannie quite well. She was really kind to me, and I liked her. She was a quiet, submissive, tiny little thing with big hair and a strong southern accent. I didn't talk to Michael's dad much, but he seemed okay . . . I guess. He mostly kept to himself. Even so, I thought Fannie was too sweet for him.

In October of '93, after four idyllic months of dating, Michael and I decided to go to Chicago together. I felt like such a grown-up taking my first vacation with a man.

We had an absolute blast! I loved showing him my city. We went to Grant Park, hit a festival, shopped downtown, and enjoyed eating at all my fave Chicago restaurants. We also went bowling with Rachel and her boyfriend at the time. *Look at me, I feel like Rachel! I'm with a beautiful man who loves me, and I'm freakishly likable.* My life seemed perfect in that moment.

After Michael and I spent the evening with Rachel, she told me the strangest thing. She said she got a bad vibe about Michael—there was something about him that she didn't trust. *Way to burst my perfect bubble.* When I asked her why, she said she wasn't sure, it was just a feeling she had. *What does she know? She doesn't know how wonderfully he treats me. She doesn't know how he kisses me. She doesn't know how he tells me he loves me every day.*

Still, her comment haunted me. Rachel would never purposely jeopardize my relationship, and she wasn't the catty or jealous type. She was a devout Catholic, a good person, and clearly smarter than me. What she said troubled me, but what was I supposed to do about a feeling she had without any probable cause?

Michael and I returned to Muskogee and continued our seemingly perfect relationship. We never argued even though we were together almost every single day. Our relationship was easy. We enjoyed each other's company and got along famously. I knew Rachel just had to be wrong.

As amazing as life was, I really missed Chicago. Muskogee had never felt like home. Michael knew this, which was why we visited Chicago. I think he was ready for a change, and he wanted to see if he loved Chicago too. He had lived in Oklahoma his entire life, and gorgeous, brilliant, educated men move to Chicago.

Ultimately, moving to Chicago didn't take much convincing because Michael had already applied at DePaul University for medical school and received an acceptance letter. Woo-hoo!

Wait.

What?

Shit.

This news was exciting for a moment, but then reality set in. I was moving to my favorite city with my favorite man, who would soon be surrounded by beautiful doctors and nurses who were much smarter than me—in a fancy school in a fancy city with fancy opportunities. My nearly two years of junior college couldn't compete with that. I figured there was absolutely no way on God's green earth I could hold on to a man of Michael's caliber.

Nevertheless, Anna was kind enough to use her connections to help us find an apartment in Chicago that would be ready in January—just in time for Michael to begin his first semester of medical school. It sounded like the perfect place, so we paid the security deposit to hold it for a couple months. Anna was going to live with us during her summer sabbaticals away from LA. That made me superexcited. Anna brought out the best in me, so that was great news.

The fall of '93 went by in a flash because time flies when living in a constant state of perfect-life bliss. By mid-October, my six-month no sex rule was nearly expired, and I was as giddy as a naughty schoolgirl. Yeah, I know what you're thinking. . . . No one waits that long to have sex. (Insert game buzzer sound here.) Wrong. Yours truly does. And surprisingly, Michael could handle the wait. Don't get me wrong—we did plenty of fun stuff up to that point, we just never had sex. By that time in my life, I'd only had sex with two men. Yes, two. No, you didn't skip a page. Did I fail to mention that I had sex with a loser named Wally? I know, I know . . . Who the hell has sex with a guy named Wally? Ding, ding, ding, ding, ding. Me. Stupid me. I have nothing nice to say about Wally. He scores a one on my personalitydar. Yep—I just made up a new word. Sorry, back to sex. Better sex. Wally, yuck.

So Michael and I had sex just before the sixth-month mark. Maybe I should've called it my five-month rule. My first time with Michael wasn't full of romance and rose petals like it was with Dante, but the actual sex was good. I'd never had an orgasm before, but with Michael, I discovered that being on top was my happy place. I couldn't be on top with Dante because my virgin body couldn't handle his enormousness. Dante, you're welcome for mentioning your huge penis in my story. Dante was Italian, which ranks high on the dickdar. Another new word. Michael was German and Irish—German below the belt—and German men fall right in the middle on the dickdar, making Michael the perfect size for my orgasmic pleasure.

By this time in my life, a sum total of maybe six weeks of my twenty-one years on the planet were sex-filled, and I felt I had some catching up to do. And catching up we did. For a good, solid, fun-filled week.

Then this happened.

NICOLE

1993

*A*s my relationship with Michael neared the six-month mark, things were perfect between us . . . or so it seemed. Again, we'd never had a single argument—not even an itty-bitty one. Then one night Michael and I were hanging out at his buddy Paul's house with a group of friends. It was really late at night, and we were drinking, smoking, and having a good time when someone started pounding on the front door. Michael casually said, "That must be Nicole." I assumed he could tell by her frantic, crazy pounding. Michael and his friends didn't even flinch—everyone just continued their conversations as if Nicole pounding madly on the door and everyone ignoring her was protocol at one o'clock in the morning at Paul's house. How did she know Michael was there? And if she cared so much, why hadn't she ever showed up at Michael's house? Did she think Michael lived with Paul?

When no one bothered to answer the door, Nicole proceeded to pound on the windows, working her way around the perimeter of the house until Michael finally went outside. I peeked out the window and saw her. She was red-haired, fiery-eyed, and—get this—extremely pregnant. Yep. Pregnant. Not just oh-look-how-cute-she's-starting-to-show pregnant. More like sit-the-fuck-down-a-baby-is-coming-any-minute-now pregnant.

Bingo! I had discovered the missing link.

That was what Rachel sensed.

That was what Paul wanted to tell me.

That was why Michael's dad never said much to me.

Well, I'd been told that Nicole had gotten pregnant and miscarried. But I never asked questions because what sensible woman wants to hear all the details about her boyfriend's ex-wife? I never went digging for information on her. That's one of the top ten ways to lose a man.

Michael came back in the house and I welcomed him with a what-the-fuck look. "Soooo, your ex-wife is, oh maybe, NINE MONTHS PREGNANT?"

"When Nicole got pregnant, I wanted to do the right thing, so I married her," he said looking sheepishly, as if he had a conscience.

"Okay." *Continue asshole.*

"Then Nicole lost the baby, but she didn't tell me, so she ended up getting pregnant again. When I found out the truth, I left. She's crazy! She's trying to trap me!"

There, there. Poor Mikey. Of course, she's crazy.

"She's violent! She hits me! She throws things at me!" he shouted as he pointed to the scar by his eye to remind me that she threw a lamp at him.

Poor baby. You're the real victim here, aren't you?

"I love you so much, and I was afraid I'd lose you. I wanted to tell you, but I thought you'd leave. I kept looking for the right moment. I'm SO sorry!"

Picture me pretending to vomit.

There I was, madly in love (and dumb as a doorknob) with a man who never willingly offered that crucial bit of information. Well, at least he didn't impregnate Nicole on my watch. We'd been together less than six months and Nicole was clearly about to burst. *Way to find the silver lining, Claire.*

So stupid, stupid, stupid me stayed with Michael. Yes, I was literally that dumb. In my defense, a person's brain doesn't fully develop until age twenty-five, and at the time, my brain was located in my vagina. My severely neglected, underutilized vagina. We'd *just* started having sex. And we were moving in together. In Chicago. And I was having orgasms. And he was hot. Like really, really hot. Okay, whatever, I was dumb as fuck.

Within a week after I found out she was pregnant, Nicole had the baby—a girl she named Abigail. Supercute name. Supercute baby. Blah, blah, blah. Michael had pictures because he actually went to the delivery room for her birth, which was the first I'd heard of Michael seeing Nicole besides that night at Paul's house.

Another week or so went by, and I woke up one morning at Michael's dad's house, went outside, and saw the words *bitch* and *whore* spray-painted all over my car. *Dumbass* would've been more accurate, but okay, whatever.

We called the police, and Michael's dad lied to them and said he saw Nicole spray-paint my car, which was totally false, but it was obviously her. Apparently, she confessed when the cops went to her house because she was ordered to pay for the damage. Just when I thought things couldn't get more awkward, Nicole and I met in a parking lot so she could give me a check. I chose a busy parking lot so she wouldn't stab me.

As I stood there in front of Nicole in the parking lot, I thought, *Wow! She's gorgeous. Like really stunning.* I'd only caught a glimpse of her outside Paul's window. She had long, straight naturally red hair and beautiful facial features. Every feature was beautiful really. I couldn't decide who was prettier between the two of us. Nicole. Yep, Nicole.

She handed me a check for half the money and said she'd pay the rest later. I was like, *Okay, that's the least I can do for screwing your ex-husband.* Looking back, I can't believe I took money from a single mom. I mean, yeah, she shouldn't have vandalized my car, but she was hormonal from the pregnancy and sad that Michael had moved on so quickly. I get it.

A few days later, Michael and I woke up to find the baby on his dad's front porch. Nicole just left Abigail there with a note saying she'd picked her up that night. Damn that baby was cute. She looked just like Michael. I wanted a superadorable, perfect-looking, Michael baby. And Michael was so endearing with her that day. I had never seen him with a baby before, but he was so gentle and attentive. Strangely enough, being a father seemed to suit him.

Shortly thereafter, Michael started spending the night with me at my parents' place—perhaps to escape all the fun surprises we'd been receiving at his dad's house. One time, in the middle of the night, Michael got off the sofa where he slept and snuck into my room. Of course, being at my parents' house, we were trying not to be so obvious that we were screwing each other every chance we got.

I was in my happy place aboard the Michael train but this particular time he, ya know, came right away. Usually, he'd slip on a condom first, but that night, he was so fast. Luckily, it was the last day of my period. A little crimson wave didn't bother Michael. *Phew. I'll be fine.*

Our quasi-perfect relationship continued. The baby surprise knocked us down a few notches, but we still never had an argument or anything, which, in hindsight, is idiotic. Finding out your boyfriend is having a baby with his ex definitely calls for an argument—a knockdown, drag-out argument. Let me just reiterate: I was twenty-one, I had an underdeveloped prefrontal cortex, and I was visiting my happy place daily. And let's face it, hot men get away with shit.

At this point, Michael and I were preparing for our upcoming move to Chicago. January was only a month away. It really should've been a gargantuan red flag that Michael was willing to leave his newborn daughter. Looking back, I'm ashamed that I didn't ax the move. I guess I thought it was Michael's choice to make, and he was so excited to start medical school. Who was I to keep a man away from his dreams (and near his ex-wife)?

SURPRISE!

LATE 1993

*I*t was Christmastime—the most wonderful time of the year. Michael and I exchanged loads of presents. He had great fashion sense, and I loved everything he picked out for me. I bought him a ton of clothes too. Expensive clothes. All Polo. I guess the gifts were appropriate for twenty-one-year-olds in love. It's not like I was expecting my ring that would take years to pay off just yet.

A few days later, I woke up and made myself a three egg, ham, and cheese omelet followed by a peanut M&M chaser. *Hmm, that's weird. I love food as much as my happy place, but I've never eaten a king-sized bag of peanut M&M's for breakfast.*

Oh.

My.

Gosh.

(Long pause to think.)

Nah.

I can't be.

Can I?

I headed out to run errands and couldn't stop thinking about my chocolate-filled breakfast. I ran into a convenience store and paced the pregnancy test aisle. I purchased the cheapest one they had.

I stuffed the test in my purse and continued to the mall where all my important errands awaited. I'm sure I had to buy something vital like lip gloss.

At the mall, I went into a department store bathroom. In the stall, there was a little metal shelf for your purse or pregnancy test or whatever. I unwrapped the pregnancy test and learned in that moment that you get what you pay for. The test was like a little chemistry experiment. Something like: take this liquid and put two drops here, then put this other liquid there, add urine here, mix this with that, do this to that, et cetera, et cetera, et cetera. Then a big purple cloud will poof into the air, and voilà! After thirty minutes and twenty-one simple steps, you'll find out whether or not you're pregnant.

Fuck.

Double fuck.

There goes my new lip gloss.

I'll never forget that moment in time. It was like my mind left my body. I walked through the entire mall (because, of course, I was nowhere near my car) in a thick haze. Everything around me was blurry and swirly. I never looked left. I never looked right. My eyes were fixated straight ahead as if I was trying to make my way through one of those spinning, whirly-twirly tunnels at a carnival. Even though I walked quickly, it felt like it took me hours to walk across the mall. When I finally arrived at my car, I had no idea how I'd even gotten there. I've never had that feeling again in my life, and hopefully, I never will.

I sat in my car for ten minutes—or all day—I'm not really sure. Somehow, I eventually managed to drive home safely.

Now what?

As usual, I was seeing Michael that night. I wondered

what he was going to do. Perhaps he would double (or triple) that engagement ring bill he'd been paying off for a year. Nothing screams Oklahoma like paying for two women's engagement rings at the same time.

I drove to Michael's work. He met me outside and had a seat in my car. *Here it goes.* When he asked me where we should go that night, I responded with four scary words: "We need to talk." I'd never said those words to him before since that's how you preface a breakup or an argument, which we'd never had.

I just came out and said it, "I'm pregnant." Done.

He just stared at me. I felt like we were having a staring contest. As I lost myself in his eyes, I didn't realize that I'd never see them again.

Our conversation ended there. He left. I went home. And I waited for him to call.

And I waited.

And I waited.

And I waited.

A few days went by, and there was still no word from him. Is this what he does to women? Impregnates them and leaves? Maybe Nicole wasn't so crazy after all. Maybe Michael deserved to be hit and have things thrown at him.

I decided to go to his dad's house. Michael wasn't home, but his dad and stepmom were. I told them I was pregnant and that Michael hadn't called me since he found out. I asked them if I could go in his room and get my stuff.

As I rummaged through Michael's things, I noticed that he hadn't taken the tags off some of his Christmas presents from me. So I took them to return, figuring I could use a couple hundred bucks.

I was about to leave, but I stopped.

I looked at Michael Sr. and Fannie and said, "Why would he leave me? We get along so well. What about

Chicago? We're supposed to move in a couple weeks! What about medical school? He's just gonna blow off an opportunity to go to DePaul Medical School? It doesn't make any sense!"

They just stared at me like I was a ghost.

"What?!" I snapped.

Blank stares continued.

"What? *What*?!" I screamed.

As Michael Sr. and Fannie took turns responding to my hysterical rant, this was what I learned that night:

Not-so-fun fact number one: Michael was actually still legally married to Nicole but supposedly only because she wouldn't sign the divorce papers. I should've left the word *whore* on my car.

Not-so-fun fact number two: Michael never once mentioned moving to Chicago to Michael Sr. or Fannie.

Not-so-fun fact number three: Michael never got accepted into DePaul Medical School. I tried to rationalize this news by telling myself that Michael never told them anything, so maybe they just didn't know. But they *did* know because . . . Wait for it. . . . Wait for it. . . .

Not-so-fun fact number four: Michael never fucking graduated from high school.

Boom.

Excuse me? Excuse me? Let me get this straight. Instead of fucking a gorgeous, brilliant, future doctor, in reality, I'm actually fucking a married, sociopathic high school dropout? And having his baby?

Okay, just making sure.

How did Michael never graduate high school when he had a reputation for being so smart and was a total bookworm? Apparently, when his parents got divorced at the end of senior year, Michael didn't take it so well. He missed the last three weeks of school, including finals. I must've been too preoccupied planning my escape route to Chicago to notice.

I went home and cried. I cried and cried and cried myself to sleep.

The next day, I told my parents over lunch.

My dad looked at me and said, "I know."

"What do you mean you know?"

My dad told me that a few weeks prior, he'd been at his desk at work when he suddenly stopped writing, set down his pen, and said to himself, "My daughter is pregnant."

My dad and I have always been close. I'm definitely a daddy's girl, so what he said didn't surprise me.

My dad suggested an abortion. Normally, he wouldn't think of abortion as the best option, but he thought it was the best decision under my circumstances. Why my dad encouraged me to have an abortion was a mystery to me. A mystery that may be solved in a couple hundred pages. No peeking.

Let me tell you a little something about my dad. He's brilliant—he's definitely the smartest being I know. He's my go-to person in life. He said he'd never trusted Michael, but he knew I would never listen. And, you're right, Dad, I wouldn't have. Somehow I've got to get my dad a sex-free, curse-free version of this book because he doesn't fall into my target audience of the dirty and open-minded. Boy, that'd be a boring book.

But my dad couldn't possibly be right about my baby. I was 100 percent certain my baby would be the best thing that ever happened to me. I wanted to document that moment as the first time my dad was wrong.

PS—When my dad said I was having a boy, I knew right then and there that I was.

Next on my list to tell: Anna.

Anna was in Chicago visiting her parents for the holidays.

I called her up bawling, and she pieced together my news in between my sobbing and nose blowing. After we hung up, I cried myself to sleep again.

The next morning, I was lying in bed and staring at the ceiling when the doorbell rang. *Who the heck is that? Maybe it's Michael stopping by to apologize. I'm so funny.*

I opened the door and there was Anna. She drove all night to come see me from Chicago. She didn't sleep one minute. That was *so* Anna.

Anna gave me the biggest hug, then we just talked and cried all day. She mentioned an abortion too. Not in a pressuring way. In an I'll-still-love-you-no-matter-what-you-decide kind of way. Anna had a gift of always knowing what to say and how to say it. And slowly but surely, her kindness rubbed off on me.

I decided not to have an abortion. I use the word *decided*, but I don't feel like that was the case exactly. I actually never entertained the idea. When two of the people I love most in the world mentioned an abortion, I physically heard the words, but I never contemplated it—not even for a moment. The second I found out I was pregnant, I felt like a mom . . . even at age twenty-one.

PREGNANCY

1994

$\mathcal{F}$rom the instant I found out I was pregnant, I took care of myself like no other twenty-one-year-old on the planet. I immediately stopped smoking and drinking. That part was easy. What was not so easy was giving up sweets and caffeine. I loved desserts as much as sex, so giving them up was a colossal sacrifice. The only dessert I allowed myself to eat was an all-natural strawberry ice cream. The kind of ice cream with three ingredients, and chocolate wasn't one of them. I ate an insane amount of fresh fruits and vegetables. Throughout my entire pregnancy, I never touched one speck of junk food. No chips, no chocolate, no cookies, no candy, no soda, no coffee, no caffeine, no fun. I did everything in my power to make a healthy baby. Looking back, I'm really impressed with my willpower and dedication at such a young age.

As amazing as I was about taking care of myself physically, I was quite the opposite about taking care of myself emotionally. Imagine going from living in Chicago and LA and all the excitement that entails to being dumped by the man you love, pregnant, and alone. Totally alone because what twenty-one-year-old wants to hang out with a pregnant chick?

Oooh, oooh, oooh, I can answer that! No one.

I went from the highest point in my life to the lowest. Like overnight. I was so sad. I had never experienced that amount of sadness. All I did was cry. I cried myself to sleep every single night. Of course, I didn't *want* to cry every night, but how do you make yourself not cry? Especially since I was heartbroken and full of pregnancy hormones.

Every night when I cried, I rubbed my belly and told my baby that I wasn't sad because of him. I told him he was the only thing that made me happy. I told him that I loved him already. I told him I'd take care of him—that we would be strong together. I told him I couldn't wait to meet him and that I would love him forever. I thought it was important to tell him that every night because I worried he felt my sadness.

I also prayed every night, just like I have my entire life. I prayed and prayed and prayed that my baby would be healthy. It's interesting, but I never prayed he'd be happy, only healthy. I think I believed *I* was the determining factor in my baby's happiness. At the time, I was taking another child psychology class. (I had enrolled for another semester of college after Michael left me.) Anyone who's ever taken a psychology class knows many psychologists believe people are a product of their environment. The whole nature versus nurture debate is one of the oldest disputes in psychology. Since I was twenty-one years old and knew absolutely everything, I was an avid believer that environmental variables were the most influential factors in shaping a child's personality, happiness, and success in life. I was definitely on the nurture side of the debate. I thought I could take any child from any background with any problem and make him (or her) happy because all children need is unconditional love and support. By that time, I was halfway finished with my degree in early childhood education. When finished, I would become a mom genius—a parenting Einstein, if you will. I'd know exactly how to make children feel valued and special. Most importantly, my son would be surrounded by love, so I knew everything would be all right.

Wrong.

I was, however, right about one thing. I knew I would be an awesome mom. After all, I was extremely dedicated to those I love. I always have been. I had also reached a time in my life that when I did things, I did them well. I even did well in school. Funnily enough, after failing high school algebra, my final grade in college algebra was 108 percent. During the entire semester, I never missed a single problem. I also got all the extra credit problems correct. The professor came up to me on the last day and shook my hand. He said no one had ever done that well in his class. Take that shitty high school algebra teacher. Apparently, *you* were the crap variable in my algebraic career. It's amazing the difference a good teacher can make. Maybe I decided to become a teacher because I had so many crappy ones.

You may have been surprised when I said I've prayed every night of my life. Perhaps you were thrown off by my potty mouth and sick sense of humor, but I consider myself a Christian. I pray a lot, actually, and feel close to God. He's my homey. I went to a Catholic church and a Catholic school in Chicago through seventh grade. Then I continued attending a Catholic church in Oklahoma for many years.

However, when I moved from Chicago to Oklahoma, I noticed a ginormous cultural difference when it came to Christianity. There are a lot of Catholics in Chicago, and—this is just my opinion, but I'm allowed to state it since this is my book—Catholics are pretty cool. It's been my experience that Catholics, particularly Catholic Chicagoans, are very down-to-earth and real. They're also fun. I know Catholic Mass is superformal and boring, but outside of church, Catholics know how to have a good time. Yes, I know I'm generalizing, so stop pointing out the obvious. Better yet, write your own book.

Oklahoma, on the other hand, was full of southern born-again Christians. Even though I was raised in the church, I had never heard of born-again Christians before moving to Oklahoma. And born-again Christians act very differently from Catholics.

Born-again Christians pray at their table before every meal—even when eating at McDonald's; Catholics pray before a family dinner at home.

Born-again Christians invite you to their church after knowing you five minutes; Catholics invite you if you say, "Hey, where do you go to church?"

Born-again Christians are charismatic, always smiling, and always in a good mood; Catholics are, I don't know, in ordinary moods.

A born-again Christian's idea of fun is a Bible–study group or a Christian rock band; Catholics have beer-filled festivals and block parties and do crazy shit like dye the Chicago River green.

Born-again Christians are extremely verbal about their faith; Catholics are more private.

Born-again Christians quote the Bible whenever they can; Catholics, um, don't.

That being said, I have almost the same beliefs as born-again Christians because, after all, theologically speaking, Catholics *are* Christians.

Let me be crystal clear that I respect all faiths and religions. I would never state that I have all the answers. That would be asinine. Oh, that reminds me, southern born-again Christians think they have all the answers.

Did I just call all southern born-again Christians asinine? No, of course not. Just all the ones I've met.

To be continued.

Michael, who will now officially be known as Sperm Donor (and was incidentally neither Catholic nor a Christian), was out of the picture, so my dad took care of me during my pregnancy. I had horrible back pain because I'd slipped a disk before my pregnancy. There were days when I could hardly stand upright because I was in so much agony. My dad rubbed my back as often as he could, which really helped. He also made sure I never missed a single Chicago Bulls game. Watching the Bulls—and salivating over Michael Jordan— was my favorite pastime. My dad would tape the games when I was at work or school so we could watch them together. For all you millennials and Generation Z'ers out there, a tape is what we used to record our shows on in order to watch them later.

When I was about eight-and-a-half-months pregnant, my dad and I went to a movie. Given my self-induced strict pregnancy diet, I had no plans to munch on popcorn or candy. I just nestled in the theater seat, trying to get my extremely pregnant self comfortable. As I sat there watching the previews, my dad ran to the restroom. When he returned, he tossed a movie-sized box of peanut M&M's on my lap. He said, "You're eating these," in a firm voice, but his eyes were smiling. Then he said, "For goodness sake, he's big enough now to handle M&M's. He wants some M&M's, dammit!" It was difficult for my dad to see me give up all my favorite things while I was pregnant, even though he knew I was doing it for my son. So there I sat, watching the movie and savoring every M&M as if I'd been reunited with chocolate after being held captive for eight months. So I guess I did have one speck of junk food while I was pregnant—one movie-sized speck. That was the happiest moment of my pregnancy—seeing a movie with my dad and eating peanut M&M's. Perhaps I should've eaten them sooner.

During the entire duration of my pregnancy, I worked, went to school full-time, and took care of myself as best I could. I just couldn't stop crying.

Every.

Single.

Night.

I cried myself to sleep.

For over eight solid months.

I still wonder if that's what went wrong.

GREYSON

1994

*A*ugust 1994 in Muskogee, Oklahoma, was sweltering hot, and I was nine months pregnant, which was about as fun as a colonoscopy. I was finishing up another semester of college over the summer. All I did was sweat, study, and sob. When I started having contractions, I frantically rallied up my parents to take me to the hospital knowing my baby would arrive promptly because that's what babies do. When we got there, I staggered through the entrance, my knees facing inward and my hands gripping my crotch, just in case my baby decided to take a nosedive into the concrete floor.

A nurse offered me pain meds and an epidural, but I refused them both. I guess I figured the last nine months weren't torturous enough. I hadn't been so careful during my pregnancy only to take drugs now. I mean, how bad could it really be?

Twenty-four hours later: "Epidural! Epidural! I'll take that epidural now!" I screamed at the nurse.

"It's too late."

"What do you mean it's too late? It's *never* too late!" No one mentioned the offer would expire.

"You're too far along now for an epidural," the nurse explained.

Yeah, yeah, yeah, I know what too late means. Fuck your time restrictions and empty uterus.

Needless to say, I did not experience an easy childbirth like some bitches do. I was in labor for twenty-four hours and pushed for two and a half. Giving birth is truly agonizing, DO NOT let anyone tell you otherwise. It's straight-up the worst pain imaginable. Men have no idea how good they have it. In addition to the unbearable pain of childbirth, there's nine months of pregnancy and twelve months of breastfeeding, times the number of babies you have. I believe there's a formula for that. It's $9x + 12x = $ fuck you.

When my son finally arrived, he didn't cry—not even a little whimper. I didn't think much of it, but it lowered his Apgar score, which is an assessment used to summarize the overall health of a newborn. He also lost a point for not exhibiting a sucking reflex and another point for being a little yellow. But, boy, was he beautiful.

I'll never forget the first moment I held him. He had huge saucerlike eyes, the cutest little nose, and a full head of hair. He was the most beautiful baby I'd ever seen. I remember grinning bigger than I'd ever smiled my entire life. My face hurt from smiling so much. I hadn't used those muscles in nine months. Then I started crying, but that time they were happy tears. I was instantly and completely in love. I named him Greyson Theodore because it sounded like a strong, professional, business name. I thought, *You can't grow up to work flippin' burgers with a name like Greyson Theodore.* Nothing against people who flip burgers. I do love a good burger.

I didn't sleep for fifty-six hours—not a single wink at the hospital. I couldn't put Greyson down. I just held him and stared at him, my heart bursting with joy. It's weird how people can tell you how much you're going to love your baby, and you think you know how much you're going to love your baby, but then you have your baby, and you're like, I never knew I could love my baby so much. You just can't fathom it until it happens.

In the hospital, two different lactation specialists tried helping me with breastfeeding, but we never had any luck. Greyson seemed incapable of sucking. The hospital gave me a contraption to stick on my nipple and a number to call if I needed additional help. Everyone seemed okay sending home a twenty-two-year-old single mom with a baby who couldn't nurse. They were like, "Too bad, so sad your baby doesn't eat. Toodles!"

PS—I didn't put Sperm Donor's name on the birth certificate.

THE NON-SLEEPING, NON-EATING, NON-CRYING NEWBORN

1994

J brought home my little bundle of joy, but nothing changed on the breastfeeding front. I put that contraption on my nipple, and it worked a tad, but not enough to get excited about. I tried feeding Greyson every hour but never had much luck. The day after I got home from the hospital, I called and made an appointment to see another lactation specialist as soon as possible. She worked with us for an hour, but Greyson just couldn't latch on. The lactation specialist recommended that I switch to formula because when we tried formula in a bottle, he was able to suck a little.

I didn't want to use formula because I was a formula-fed baby and suffered extremely severe earaches my entire childhood. I was also never the quickest bunny in the forest. I read that breastfeeding increases brain development, decreases earaches and respiratory illnesses, strengthens the immune system, and promotes bonding—so I had my heart set on breastfeeding. Plus, breastfeeding helped with postpartum weight loss, and I no longer had a perfect body.

I immediately made an appointment with a fourth

lactation specialist, but nothing changed. Greyson continued getting a little milk with the contraption, but not enough. I supplemented with formula a bit to buy me some time. He was losing weight, which is normal for a newborn, but I had to act quickly. I was also told that if he was hungry, he'd cry. But he never did.

I spoke to my neighbor across the street about my breastfeeding problem. She had four children, and I used to cut all their hair for free. For some odd reason, I was really good at cutting hair with absolutely no formal training. Anyway, she gave me her breast pump. I know it seems a little gross to use someone else's breast pump, but it was nothing a little boiling water couldn't fix.

I don't even know if they had fancy electric breast pumps in 1994, but whatever the opposite of a fancy electric breast pump is, that's what she gave me. It was a small, handheld, manual breast pump. It worked well, but it took me forever to pump. So this was how I spent my days: When Greyson was awake, I held him and smothered him with kisses. When Greyson was asleep, I pumped my boobs. I pumped about four hours a day—fifteen minutes here, fifteen minutes there —during Greyson's annoyingly brief, sporadic naps. That's how important breastfeeding was to me.

The good news was that Greyson was finally getting enough breast milk. The bad news was that I had to feed him with a bottle since it was the only thing he could latch onto. Kinda. He continued to struggle, so feeding him took a ton of patience.

Greyson also hardly napped during the day, yet he still managed not to sleep a wink at night. Keeping me up all day and night was Greyson's favorite. I thought babies were supposed to sleep a lot. Not Greyson. For months, I just walked around the house like a zombie carrying him all night long. If I set him down, he grunted and flopped around like a fish out of water. At least when I held him, he was calm and would sleep a little. I never knew what exhaustion was until I had Greyson. People warned me that I'd never sleep after the baby was born. In my head, I scoffed at them, thinking that I knew what it was like to never sleep. But after Greyson was born, I realized that I never knew what not sleeping was actually like.

Greyson eventually began sleeping at night, but he never slept *through* the night. He woke up every single hour, every single night. Grunt, flop, grunt, flop, grunt, flop, until I picked him up.

For.

Eighteen.

Solid.

Months.

That is not an exaggeration. I literally did not sleep for eighteen months. I know I'm totally skipping ahead here, but I want you to wrap your brain around the fact that I, an actual living human, did not sleep for more than an hour at a time for eighteen months. Autographs later.

Greyson had a crib, and I had every intention of using it, but with his brutal eating and sleeping difficulties, I slept next to him instead. I loved looking at him and cuddling him when he slept. I had read the book *The Family Bed*, which encouraged sleeping next to your baby. The philosophy outlined in the book seemed best for Greyson and me at the time. Since then, I have changed my opinion on sleeping with a baby, but I strongly respect all parents who do what they believe is best for their child. All children and families are different, so I would never say one way is better than another.

So, in a nutshell, Greyson was a terrible eater, a terrible sleeper, but he never, ever cried. He never cried for even one second. Ever. I took Greyson to a neurologist and told him that he'd literally never cried. The doctor asked some questions, did some basic tests, and said I was taking too good of care of him so he never had a reason to cry.

Hmm, well, that was true. I read that you can't spoil a baby, so I cuddled, rocked, and played with him every second of the day unless I was at school. I was no longer working, but I did start taking classes again when Greyson was a few weeks old. I scheduled my classes at night so my working parents could watch him while I went to school three nights a week. I did all my homework at night while Greyson slept —in one-hour increments.

When Greyson was two months old, he was baptized. It just so happened that his baptism landed on Dante's and Ben's birthdays—October 2. A fabulous reminder of the mentally sound, non-sociopathic, normal men I'd loved and lost. And, apparently, I had a thing for Libras. I certainly didn't plan that date, but it was the only available Sunday at our church that worked for everyone involved.

Anna and my brother flew to Oklahoma to be Greyson's godparents. Anna was born and raised Catholic. I'm pretty sure being a cool godmother isn't a requirement of the Catholic Church, but I knew Anna would be just that. Buying nice presents was also not a prerequisite of godmotherhood, but I knew she'd do that too. Anna was the most generous person I'd ever known. As soon as Greyson was born, she sent him a gigantic stuffed dog from FAO Schwarz. In the '90s, FAO Schwarz was posh and extremely expensive. Anna spent an insane amount on that dog, but that was typical Anna. However, that's not why I picked Anna to be Greyson's godmother. I picked Anna because she was a dedicated Catholic, and I knew she would always be there for Greyson and me. And I knew she would play an integral role in Greyson's life and upbringing.

Anna always talked about how once she became famous

she would move us to LA and help me with Greyson. If anyone else would've said that, I would've been like, "Whatevs." But when Anna said it, I knew she meant it with all her heart. I had this image of life in LA with my movie star best friend. Anna was going to change the world, and I would be her Gayle King.

MY LITTLE JOKESTER

1995

*I*t was January 1995, and Greyson was five months old. I was still pumping four hours a day because he wouldn't nurse, waking up every hour of the night because he wouldn't sleep, and wondering why he seemed to be the only baby in the universe who didn't cry.

As fun as it was pumping four hours a day, I decided to give a fifth lactation specialist a shot. She came to my house and worked diligently with us. She taught me to put my pointer finger upside down in Greyson's mouth, so the pad of my finger rested on the roof of his mouth. She said to do that all day, every day, to help Greyson practice and strengthen his sucking.

I stuck my finger in that boy's mouth every day until my finger looked like a shriveled-up prune. Then, hallelujah, Greyson finally learned to nurse, and I got about thirty hours a week of my life back when I was able to stop pumping.

Greyson may have learned to nurse, but he was past the age of when he should've learned to smile. Babies typically smile by two or three months old, but Greyson never did. I played peekaboo, sang silly songs, kissed his little toes—anything to make him smile—but I got nothing. I called him, in my deepest voice, "My very serious baby." With a very staid look on his face, he'd just look around like he was thinking. He was like a pint-sized CEO.

Another thing Greyson was very behind on was making eye contact. Most babies begin making eye contact by two or three months of age. I always made a conscious effort to try to look Greyson in the eyes, but even when his face was physically turned toward my face, his eyes would look sharply to the side. Then when I would move into his line of vision, his eyes immediately flipped to the opposite side. It was like he was playing a game with me. At five months old, Greyson purposely avoided eye contact.

Bonding with Greyson and exposing him to stimulating environments were very important to me. I tried to get him out of the house as much as possible. My aunt sent me the greatest baby sling, and everywhere I went, I carried Greyson in it. I loved it because it comfortably put Greyson on my chest at the perfect height for lots of kisses. I could also talk to him easily while we walked around the park, the mall, the zoo—everywhere. I liked that he was always close to me.

When Greyson was a baby, I joined a wonderful program for single moms. As part of the free program, a child-development specialist came to my house every month for a year to assess Greyson's fine and gross motor (physical) skills and cognitive (intellectual) development. I loved when she came over because she was in awe of Greyson. Greyson was just average with his fine and gross motor skills, but cognitively, he blew her away. She always said things like, "I've never seen a baby understand object permanence this early." Then a couple months later, "I've never seen a baby complete a puzzle this early." Greyson hit cognitive milestones months, sometimes even years, in advance. I felt so proud.

Even though Greyson was showing early signs of extreme intelligence, he was beginning to do something troubling: his arms flailed around as if he was trying to hit me. When he did that, I would gently hold his arms for a moment and say, "Your arms are for hugging, not hitting," but he continued to hit me repeatedly. I had never read about babies hitting or studied anything about it in all my early childhood education classes. Remember, this was in 1994, BC (Before Computers), so the average person didn't own a computer or have Internet access. In other words, this information was not at my fingertips.

Speaking of nonexistent things, I decided to reach out to Sperm Donor's family. Surely Fannie and Michael Sr. would be interested in seeing their grandson, right? I mean, gee whiz, it wasn't their fault that Sperm Donor blatantly played a game with my life, lied about every aspect of our relationship, and left me to raise his son by myself. So I thought I'd show them my gorgeous son, and, of course, they'd fall in love with him and want to be in his life forever —because that's what humans do.

Fannie showed a little interest, but technically she wasn't related to Greyson since she was Sperm Donor's stepmother. I decided to pursue a relationship with her anyway because maybe it would lead to the rest of Sperm Donor's family getting involved. Plus, I was hoping she would tell Sperm Donor how good I looked because I looked fucking fantastic. Breastfeeding worked wonders because I was eating nonstop and down to a size 3. I was actually thinner than I was *before* I got pregnant with Greyson, even though I gained forty pounds during my pregnancy. Being young helped, but breastfeeding played a big part in getting my body back. My hair was also really long, blonde, and healthy. That was the best I ever looked in my life. Everywhere I went, I could feel men staring at me—not asking me out with a baby in tow, but they definitely checked me out. A lot.

I set up a time to meet with Fannie. When we met, she tried to get a good look at Greyson, but he kept turning away like he always did when someone tried to look in his eyes. So she walked to the other side, but he turned his head again. Fannie went back and forth, back and forth for a few minutes. Then she was like, "Why won't he let me look at him?" I laughed and said, "He's such a jokester," but inside I knew that wasn't true.

After that, I spoke to Fannie every now and then, but nothing materialized. Michael Sr. continued to show absolutely no interest in Greyson. I'd never met Sperm Donor's mom or sister, so I wasn't sure what to do about them. I knew Sperm Donor's mom lived in Texas, but that was it. Certainly, if they wanted to, any of them could easily find Greyson and me living with my parents in the same house I'd lived in since eighth grade. Sperm Donor's family's lack of interest in Greyson made me feel like I'd made the right decision not putting his name on Greyson's birth certificate. I also decided not to sue Sperm Donor for child support. I honestly believed he would eventually grow up and want to contribute financially or otherwise. It seemed unfathomable to me that a man could have a son and never want to help. Boy, did he prove me wrong over twenty years and zero dollars later.

Greyson was missing one side of his family, but my family made up for it. My parents were so in love with Greyson and were extremely attentive and loving grandparents. When I wasn't cuddling or playing with Greyson, my parents were. They also helped me out financially so Greyson didn't have to go to day care. They wanted him to have the best possible childhood. Even though they wished I'd had a baby under different circumstances, they were crazy about Greyson. I can confidently say no baby was more loved in the world. The three of us were totally smitten with him.

WHAT TO DO WHEN YOUR BABY
ATTACKS YOU

1995

*W*hen Greyson was six months old, I took him to the doctor for a checkup. His pediatrician had wooden paddles hanging on the wall in every room so parents could use them to discipline their children because apparently going to the doctor wasn't frightening enough. This was (and I believe still is) quite common in the South where they have a born-again Christian spare-the-rod-spoil-the-child mentality.

Related, unrelated story: Back when I was in high school in Muskogee, the principal had a wooden paddle hanging on the wall of his office. Three times, I got caught breaking the rules—once I lost my gym locker combination and twice I wore a non-cheerleading miniskirt that was too short. As punishment, I had a choice between swats or detention. But it wasn't really a choice because I had either dance or cheer practice every day before and after school when detention was held, and if I missed practice, I got demerits and couldn't perform. So all three times I "chose" swats. When I went to the principal's office, he closed the door and made me put my elbows on his desk—putting my cute, perky, miniskirt-wearing ass up in the air. He then took his wooden paddle and swatted me a couple times. Hard. Really hard. Like unable-to-sit-when-I-returned-to-class hard. It's funny that in all my years in Catholic school in Chicago, I never witnessed—or even heard about—a nun hitting a student with a ruler like the stereotype suggests. But throw me in a public school in Oklahoma and there was a man with a boner swatting the shit out of my perfect little ass in his private office. I know my readers from the South are probably thinking, *Yeah, so what?* and my readers from everywhere else are probably thinking, *Are you f'ing kidding me?!* Google "corporal punishment in public schools," and you'll see that this is still happening in several states. I'm just pointing out the vast cultural and religious differences within our country. Now back to Greyson's paddle-pushing pediatrician.

I told the pediatrician Greyson didn't cry, make eye contact, smile, or sleep, and that he'd just learned to nurse and hit me constantly throughout the day. Then I finally said these words out loud, "I think Greyson is autistic." He said there was no way I could tell at six months old.

Putz. I had known for months.

Back in 1994, the year Greyson was born, no one talked about autism. The word *autism* was exclusively associated with Dustin Hoffman's character in the movie *Rain Man*. I had never met, heard of, or seen anyone with autism before, but I'd learned about it in my early childhood education classes. I was also pretty intuitive—except when it came to men, clearly. I knew Greyson had autism, but I also knew there was something very unique about him. I felt in my heart that God gave me an extraordinary child, and He chose me to raise him. I felt like the luckiest mom in the world.

Between the ages of six and twelve months old, Greyson continued to hit me—about a hundred times a day, every single day. No, that's not a typo, he actually hit me about a hundred times a day.

The smallest instance would trigger a hitting fit—like if Greyson tried putting something dangerous in his mouth and I took it away. Without warning, Greyson would violently flail his arms at me—often smacking my nose, pulling out a chunk of my hair, scratching my face, or whacking my teeth. During these episodes, Greyson's eyes and face looked unresponsive, like Greyson wasn't really there. His eyes stared forward and his face went . . . blank. I would gently hold down his arms and speak softly, hoping to settle him down. But the instant I let go of his arms, he would go right back to violently flailing them at me. So I'd hold his arms down again for about ten minutes. I would hum, sing a song, or rock him—anything to calm him down. Then, once he seemed settled, I would let go again. He'd thrash his arms at me like I never did anything to calm him. As crazy as it sounds, I swear it seemed like he tried to trick me by acting calm so I'd let go just so he could hit me some more. But that's silly, a baby can't outwit me . . . I think.

So he'd hit me, I'd hold him, he'd settle, I'd let go.

Hit, hold, settle, let go.

Hit, hold, settle, let go.

Finally, after about forty-five minutes, he'd just snap out of it and suddenly become Greyson again like nothing had ever happened.

Because Greyson was still a baby, I didn't have many options on how to handle his hitting fits. You can't reason with a six-month-old, put them in a time-out, or send them to their room, and I didn't really believe in spanking, particularly a baby. Plus, it seemed counterproductive to try to teach a baby not to hit by hitting.

When Greyson and I were out, his episodes lessened. I believe it was because his mind was busy soaking up all the stimulation. But when it did happen, it was humiliating. Sometimes he had episodes when I took him to the park and swing time was over. I would carry him to the car while he attacked me. I felt the moms staring at me with disapproval and imagined what they were saying to one another. "She must be a horrible mother not being able to control her baby," the mom of the baby who giggled in the swing would say. "She must beat her baby! How else would a baby learn to beat his mom?" her friend with the toddler who gleefully went down the slide would reply.

I bet their children smiled and made eye contact at three months old.

Once, Greyson had an episode at the mall. I'll never forget how it felt carrying a baby through an entire mall while he hit me hundreds of times. I couldn't keep his arms down as I carried him, so he just beat me up as I scurried through the mall mortified. I saw the looks of judgment on everyone's faces, like I was walking through a tunnel of persecuting eyes. No one in that mall knew what a dedicated mom I was. No one in that mall had a baby who hit them like that every day. No one in that mall loved their child more than I loved Greyson.

Ever since that day, when I see a mom with a toddler having a tantrum, I try to say something to make her feel like she's not alone, "I sure don't miss those days! Hang in there!"

When Greyson wasn't having an episode, he was actually quite wonderful. Of course, he never cried, so that was a weird bonus. And at this point, he was nursing well too. He still woke up every hour, but other than never sleeping or smiling and beating me every day, he was a very pleasant baby. He was always exploring and looked deep in thought. I felt like Greyson was an old soul trapped in a baby's body— like he was just frustrated because his mental self wasn't aligned with his physical self. It was as if he was too young to vocalize his thoughts, do what he wanted to do, and go where he wanted to go. Like his body had to catch up with his wisdom. Looking at Greyson that way helped me comprehend his episodes. Logical or not, I couldn't think of another explanation since his behaviors weren't covered in any of my early childhood education courses. And in all the books I read, there were no chapters titled, "What to Do When Your Baby Attacks You."

Life was extremely challenging as a single mom, but it was also very lonely. I went from a life full of fun and excitement to a life full of breastfeeding, changing diapers, and sleepless nights. From a life full of bars and concerts to a life full of baby swings and wagon rides. From a life full of friends and men to a life full of Greyson, Greyson, Greyson. I never went out with friends because, oh yeah, no one wanted to hang out with a friend with a baby. Which meant I had no friends except Rachel in Chicago and Anna in Los Angeles. I felt sad, alone, and stuck in Oklahoma. I was in the prime of my life, and I spent it without friends or men.

I decided to lift my spirits by going to Chicago for a couple weeks during the summer in 1995. I drove there with Greyson when he was ten months old. Of course, Rachel's parents let Greyson and me stay with them. We even went to Lake Geneva where we spent our days on the beach and our nights grilling and laughing. I don't remember asking Rachel's parents back then if I could stay with them every summer for a decade. But I did. I just showed up—like a herpes outbreak. Yet they never made me feel unwelcome. Thank you Rachel's parents for making me feel like family for so many years. I'd love to say to my younger entitled self and any entitled readers out there that nobody owes you anything. When someone helps you or welcomes you into their home, just know that you're an inconvenience, so be appreciative and thankful.

That summer, Greyson and I also spent some time with Anna since she returned to Chicago every summer. We spent our days shopping or at the beach. It was just like the good ol' days—minus the bars, the parties, the dancing, the men, the drinks, and all the excitement. But at least it was nice being with Anna again. I felt a flicker of myself come back until I had to return to Oklahoma where my soul was sucked out of my body and run over by a pickup truck.

JESUS CHRIST IS IN THE HOUZZZZ

1995–1996

$\mathcal{W}$hen I was twenty-three, I decided to explore different beliefs and religions. I'd been Catholic my entire life, so I didn't know much about other religions or much about that born-again Christian business. I'd met a lot of born-again Christians and often wondered why they were always smiling. It was so damn irritating.

I wanted to make sure that I raised Greyson according to *my* beliefs, not just the only beliefs I'd ever known. So I started reading books about Buddhism, Judaism, Hinduism, and Christianity. And for the first time in my life, I decided to visit a church that wasn't Catholic.

I pulled up to a born-again Christian church on a Friday night because that's how the born-again Christian churches roll in Muskogee. It was also foreign to me that the "church" was located in a high school auditorium. *I guess when I'm bored I'll gaze at a maroon and gold cougar on the cement block wall instead of stained glass and oil paintings of Christ.*

When I arrived at the high school, I mean church, there were an insane number of cars trying to park, so volunteers were directing traffic. In Chicago, they did that at my fave burger joint, but never at a church. The number of cars surpassed the number of parking spots, so I had to park in a dirt field. As I hesitantly stepped out of my car with Greyson, I was startled to hear someone blow a whistle and scream into a megaphone, "Kid here! Kid here!," which made me wonder if they'd ever seen a kid before. Within thirty seconds, a volunteer with a wheelbarrow ran up and said, "Your son's ride ma'am." *Well, all righty then.* I tossed, or gently placed, Greyson in the wheelbarrow, and the volunteer rolled him to the entrance. I can safely say that no Catholic church offers wheelbarrow rides to the door. I kinda dug it.

Greyson and I strolled through the door wearing our Sunday best (even though it was Friday) only to realize that almost everyone around us was wearing shorts and flip-flops. Several people had Big Gulps in hand. I kinda dug that too.

As we made our way down the hall, I noticed everyone gathering around a table. *Hmm, what's on the table? Collection basket? Church programs? Holy water? The body of Christ? Nope.* On the table sat a giant bowl of candy. And not just Tootsie Rolls, real candy. *That's it, I've decided that I'm now a born-again Christian.* I grabbed some peanut M&M's to get me through what I predicted to be a very long and tedious service.

I dropped Greyson off at Sunday school—correction, Friday night school—and prayed the beeper I was handed wouldn't buzz during the service. My stomach was in knots as the teacher explained that I should retrieve Greyson if they buzzed me. As I nervously looked for a seat in the auditorium, I reminded myself that Greyson's behavior was better when he was out of the house and in a stimulating environment.

Once I got settled, the band started playing some upbeat, really loud, actually not bad, Christian rock music. *Shouldn't an eighty-year-old woman be playing the organ and leading a hymn?* Everyone started dancing at their seats. *Um, excuse me everyone, just a heads-up, I'm pretty sure we're supposed to be kneeling silently with our heads bowed.* After ten minutes of surprisingly good music, out walked the pastor. The very attractive pastor. *Pure thoughts, pure thoughts, pure thoughts.* It was really hard to remember that I was at church. And then, Attractive Pastor began to speak. Intelligently. Charismatically. Hilariously. That hot—I mean that God-fearing—man could speak! I'd never been so engaged at a church in my life. Come to think of it, I'd never been engaged at church at all. Usually, by that time in a service, I was finished perusing the family pictures in the church directory and on to counting the pews for the fifth time. But instead, I was listening—wholeheartedly listening. Hanging on every word and not because he was attractive, although that helped, but because he was fantastic. It was like JC was in the houzzzz! Jesus Christ, Jim Carrey, you pick. He made me laugh. He made me cry. He took biblical stories and related them to everyday life in a heartfelt, hilarious way. *This born-again Christian thing isn't half bad.*

Not only did I have a new church, I also had a new degree. In May 1996, I graduated with a Bachelor of Science degree in early childhood education. (Insert firecrackers here.) I graduated college cum laude, by the way, which is shocking news for anyone who knew me in high school. I was finally equipped to provide for my son as a single mom. Until that point of motherhood, I lived with my parents, and they supported Greyson and me financially, and for that, I will be forever grateful. If not for my parents, Greyson would have been in day care full-time while I worked and went to school. Emotionally, I could not have handled leaving Greyson every day. Greyson staying with my loving parents so I could go to class at night was difficult enough. I can't imagine how difficult leaving him at day care would've been.

Even with my new diploma, my mind seemed inferior to Greyson's. Cognitively, he was growing by leaps and bounds. He loved doing puzzles. One of his favorite things to do as a one-year-old was to make a giant circle of about twelve wooden puzzles around him. Then he'd take the puzzles, dump all the pieces into a pile in the middle of the circle where he sat, and return each wooden base back to its spot in the circle. Then he'd complete all twelve puzzles at once by grabbing random pieces from the pile. My father and I watched him in awe. When Greyson faced the opposite direction in the circle, my dad sometimes took two pieces and swapped their spots. As soon as Greyson turned around, he would immediately spot the wrong pieces and fix them without skipping a beat. All of his puzzles were labeled for ages three or higher, so I knew that was remarkable for a one-year-old. Greyson always did things that fascinated me.

One of his favorite wooden puzzles was an alphabet puzzle. When he did that puzzle, I sat with him and said each letter as he placed it in the puzzle. I never thought much of it until he started saying the letters before me. Greyson hardly spoke, but he could identify every single letter in the alphabet. I knew Greyson was smart, but when he did that, it confirmed that I was given a unique and spectacular child.

Greyson drew a lot of attention to us that ranged from astonishment to disgust. We had zoo passes, so we went once a week. One day we were sitting on the train ride at the zoo. Every seat had a sign that posted the train's rules. "Warning: Please keep all hands and feet inside the train." I was sitting with Greyson, waiting for the train to leave, and a five-year-old boy was sitting behind us with his mom. Greyson overheard the boy trying to name all the letters on the sign.

His mom lovingly encouraged him as he struggled through the letters.

When Greyson heard the boy struggling, he pointed to the sign and quickly recited each letter, "W-A-R-N-I-N-G-P-L-E-A-S-E-K-E-E-P-A-L-L-H-A-N-D-S-A-N-D-F-E-E-T-I-N-S-I-D-E-T-H-E-T-R-A-I-N," then looked at the boy as if to say, "How can you not know that?"

"Greyson, aren't you excited to go on the train?" I said excitedly, trying to change the subject.

Greyson responded, "W-A-R-N-I-N-G-P-L-E-A-S-E-K-E-E-P-A-L-L-H-A-N-D-S-A-N-D-F-E-E-T-I-N-S-I-D-E-T-H-E-T-R-A-I-N."

The mom behind me asked, "Excuse me, how old is your son?"

I hesitantly responded, "Um, one."

And there was the look—like a deer in headlights. *When's this train leaving anyway? Maybe that lady will see Greyson beat me up later when it's time to leave the monkey house. That'll make her feel better.*

Yes, Greyson was still hitting me on a daily basis. "Hit me" was really an endearing way to put it; "beat the shit out of me" was much more accurate because he never just hit me once. When I upset him, he hit me and hit me and hit me and hit me. For forty-five solid minutes. If an adult hits another adult a hundred times, it's aggravated assault. Or murder. Greyson's episodes, mixed with his brilliance, made raising him very confusing. My feelings wavered between being proud, being flabbergasted, and being scared.

But at least I was no longer exhausted. Greyson finally learned to sleep through the night at eighteen months old. I attributed his horrible sleep habits to how smart he was—like he had a hard time shutting down his brain. He wanted to learn every possible second of the day and didn't want to miss anything. I could tell by the way he examined everything that his mind never stopped. He was like a tiny little mad scientist.

However, Greyson still never naturally smiled. The only time he smiled was when I made him laugh by tickling him. When I wanted to take a picture of him, I couldn't just tell him to smile or say cheese or even catch him smiling—which was too bad because Greyson was so darling with his saucerlike eyes, button nose, and blond hair. To get a picture, I put my camera in one hand and tickled him with the other hand. Then if I was fast enough, I would get a picture of him smiling. Never once did Greyson just smile at someone or smile out of happiness. He only had two looks—deep in thought and, well, sad. He always looked sad. There were no digital cameras back then, so I threw out thousands of pictures of Greyson looking sad. Thinking ahead to when he was an adult, I didn't want him to look at his baby album and say, "Boy, I sure look miserable." Plus, I needed happyish pictures to show his future wife.

By this time in our lives, Rachel, my childhood bestie, had found her Prince Charming—a man as adorable and hilarious as her, if that's even possible. During the summer of 1996, Rachel was getting married, so I drove to Chicago with my parents, and they watched Greyson while I served as a bridesmaid in Rachel's wedding. I was pissed that I wasn't chosen to be her maid of honor, especially since we'd made a pact in fourth grade that she'd let me be her maid of honor in exchange for the last green olive in the jar we were sharing. *How dare she choose her sister and break our Green Olive Pact!* I assumed Rachel getting married put an end to me staying at her parents' house uninvited for an undisclosed amount of time. I think? Not sure.

It was a good thing I had Anna as a replacement best

friend because I knew I'd soon become a distant memory for Rachel. She always seemed to put me on the back burner when she had a boyfriend, so I was doomed with her having a husband. Anna was never like that. She didn't have time for men, so I knew Anna and I would be best friends forever.

ALLISON, ANNA, AND AIDS

1996–1997

$\mathcal{I}$ decided to break in my new degree and work part-time. When Greyson was two, I got a job at an elementary school as an after-school art teacher. It was the perfect job for me because I only worked from three to six, Monday through Friday. My mom was home from work by then because she taught at an alternative middle school with really early hours. Greyson also kinda sorta napped every day around three. I've always really enjoyed art, so it was a great job at the time.

By the time I'd been at my new job a couple weeks, I'd turned the art area into the most popular part of the after-school program. I had to create a sign-up sheet because so many kids wanted to be at my station. Even though I worked until six, most of the students were picked up by five, so during the last hour, I played games and did puzzles with the few kids who were always picked up last. All the kids were great, but I grew especially fond of one particular girl named Allison. She was extremely shy and timid, so she didn't interact with the other kids a lot. She was supercute with long red hair and freckles and was always dressed adorably.

Her grandmother picked her up every day at six o'clock sharp. We often exchanged pleasantries, and I'd tell her I thought her granddaughter was very sweet. I heard from other teachers that Grandma had full custody and was raising Allison.

As the school year went by, I enjoyed getting to know Allison and the other students. My boss liked me because I was reliable, superorganized, and did great art projects. This was back when the Internet was a new thing, so there was no Google and no Pinterest. I got ideas from books or my own brain. My art projects were done on cave walls or chiseled in stone. Just kidding; I'm not *that* old!

One day I was busy cleaning the art area when I looked up and saw someone I never expected to see again. It was Nicole—yes, *that* Nicole—the woman who used to throw things at Sperm Donor. *What the hell is Nicole doing here?* I pretended to pick up scraps off the floor behind the art table and watched her walk across the room toward Allison, who yelled, "Mommy!" and they walked out the door.

No freakin' way. I was not expecting that. My heart was pounding out of my chest as I tried to make sense of it in my head. Well, the red hair added up. That's one. Sperm Donor never talked about Nicole, so I was positive he'd never mentioned that she had another daughter. Allison was six years old, so Nicole must have had her right after high school. *Whoa!*

After that day, I continued to treat Allison as if I'd never received that tidbit of information. It certainly wasn't Allison's fault that the adults around her were a mess, including yours truly. I felt sad that Nicole wasn't raising Allison but was raising her little sister, Abigail—at least as far as I knew. It must have been heartbreaking for Allison knowing that her mom kept Abigail, but not her. On the other hand, Allison's grandma was lovely and took such good care of her. That was obvious from Allison's fancy clothes with matching hair bows and the way Grandma interacted with her at pickup time each day. So maybe Nicole thought Grandma was the best decision for Allison. Nicole had gone through a lot—first she'd had Allison so young with Asshole Number One, then she'd had a baby with Asshole Number Two (aka Michael) who'd left her. That's a lot of pain to go through. I knew firsthand what the latter felt like. I wished the best for Nicole, Allison, and Abigail. But not Sperm Donor. He can suck it.

Toward the end of the school year, Allison's grandma, who still didn't know who I was, approached me. She said that Allison normally had a really hard time opening up to people and trusting them, but she really liked me. Then she asked me if I'd be interested in being Allison's nanny over the summer.

Um, how can I put this? . . . No.

She proceeded to give me her phone number and asked me to think about it and give her a call. *Yep, sure thing. I'll do that. Think about it. Nicole would seriously have a heart attack. First, I unintentionally steal her husband, then, I unintentionally steal her daughter. That would go over really well.*

After a few days, I gave Allison's grandmother a call and told her the truth—that I was the woman who ruined (or saved) her daughter's life. I told her I was the mom of her *other* granddaughter's half brother. *All y'all non-rednecks out there take un momento to think 'bout dat. I can't make this shit up.*

Shockingly, Allison's grandmother still wanted me to be her nanny. I told her I wouldn't feel right taking on that role unless Nicole said it was okay, which, of course, she wouldn't.

Grandma later told me that she'd already spoken with Nicole. Then—probably after needing to be resuscitated, Nicole muttered, "No way in hell."

Grandma had to find a different nanny for Allison, and I had to find a different job. That was way too Oklahoma for me.

With all that hillbilly drama, I was so happy to get a call from my Hollywood bestie, Anna. I couldn't wait to tell her that my favorite student was Sperm Donor's ex-wife's daughter. Anna was my bright, shiny light at the end of my Oklahoma tunnel of doom. She was the person who helped me see the bigger picture and made me feel like everything would be okay.

Until it wasn't.

When she called me, she said four horrible words, "We have to talk."

I got a pit in my stomach. I'd never heard Anna sound so serious. "Are you pregnant?"

"I wish."

Oh no, it must be bad. Anna didn't want kids until after she won her first Oscar, so she'd never wish to be pregnant.

Silence fell on the line.

"I have AIDS," she whispered.

"What? I can't hear you." *Or at least I certainly didn't hear you correctly.*

"I have AIDS," she repeated.

"That's impossible. That's impossible," I whispered.

"William. I got it from William," she mumbled.

"Are you sure?"

"I had a routine blood test and abnormalities showed up. They tested me for HIV, and it came back positive. They made me do it twice because the doctors didn't believe it."

"I don't know what to say. I'll come see you."

"You can't. I left my apartment in Los Angeles, and I'm home with my parents. Now is not a good time. You take care of Greyson."

We both just cried on the phone. I was too shocked to speak. That was the worst phone call of my life.

I didn't understand. In the mid-90s supposedly only gay men and heroin addicts got AIDS. It made absolutely no sense that a straight woman who never did so much as smoke a cigarette or get drunk and who'd only ever slept with one man her entire life had contracted the AIDS virus. The most kind, tenacious, genuine, humble, loyal, ethical, strong, likable person I ever knew my entire life had contracted the AIDS virus.

What.

The.

FUCK!

The world as I knew it was replaced with nothingness.

A couple months went by, and I drove with Greyson to Chicago to visit Anna. When I saw her I gave her the biggest hug and didn't want to let go. When our eyes met, she must've seen sorrow because all she said to me was "Don't." So we went on with our day as if that horrible phone call had never happened.

We enjoyed a day at the zoo, where I tried my damnedest not to stare at Anna and look for signs of AIDS. She looked like the same Anna. She acted like the same Anna. She smiled like the same Anna. My eyes saw the same healthy and beautiful Anna. My brain wondered how she had unknowingly had the virus for years. My heart felt heavy and helpless.

We then went to a restaurant where Anna attempted to have a conversation with Greyson. She'd interacted with him at the zoo, but that was more like "look at the lion" and "look at that monkey swinging," veering Greyson's attention away from her instead toward her. But at the restaurant, she kept trying to make eye contact with Greyson. His eyes looked off to the side like they always did when someone tried to look at him. I knew she could tell something was wrong, but Anna would never say anything to make me sad. Anna knew that I knew she knew and that was good enough. We had an unspoken understanding: an understanding not to talk about what was wrong with Greyson or about AIDS.

Later that night, I discovered I had a few mosquito bites. Back in the '90s, there were still a lot of questions about AIDS, so the mosquito bites terrified me. I frantically searched every inch of Greyson's body for bites, but fortunately, he had none. That night I called the hotline 1-800-AID-AIDS and asked if I could contract HIV through a mosquito bite. The man on the line said there were no documented cases of someone contracting HIV through a mosquito bite. I hung up and called back hoping for a more concrete answer. Again and again and again. Well, that didn't make me feel better at all. I never got the concrete "that's impossible" I was looking for. To me it made perfect sense that if a mosquito sucked blood out of Anna and then thirty seconds later sucked blood out of me, I would become infected. I didn't sleep that night. I just kept contemplating over and over in my head the likelihood of the same mosquito biting Anna and then biting me.

The next day I met Anna in downtown Chicago. We had a fun day planned to shop and go to the beach. I bought some bug spray before meeting her and sprayed the heck out of Greyson and me. I obviously didn't mention my mental state or exhaustion and just tried to enjoy the day. I brought Greyson's umbrella stroller with me because I knew we'd do a lot of walking. It was a cheap, crappy little umbrella stroller. You know, the kind a single mom with no child support would own. I hated that stroller and hardly used it back home. It had a sharp piece of plastic on the side of the handle that stuck out, and I'd cut my hand on it a couple times in the past.

I was pushing Greyson around downtown Chicago, having a good time shopping with Anna. She wanted to help with Greyson, so she occasionally pushed the stroller for me. At one point during the day, I heard Anna say, "Ouch!" Well, of course, she'd scraped her hand on that stupid piece of plastic because I forgot to tell her to watch out for it. I wanted to inspect her hand and see how deeply she'd scraped it, but I didn't want it to be obvious that I was checking for blood. Instead, I was just careful not to cut my hand. I felt on edge all day about that damn stroller.

We headed to the beach so Greyson could play in the sand. Greyson was having a great time with Anna. She was very engaging and attentive to Greyson. We made a sandcastle and decorated it with rocks. We were all having a lovely time, successfully pretending life was great. Anna told me she was excited to go back to Los Angeles to work. Of course she was.

After a couple hours of playing in the sand, we decided to head to dinner. Anna grabbed Greyson's hand and ran with him through the sand. Both of them were barefoot and Anna pretended to run in slow motion, being goofy to entertain Greyson, but of course, he never cracked a smile. She picked him up and swung him around. Still, nothing. She was probably checking to see if Greyson was capable of smiling. Which, of course, he was not. As she ran through the sand holding Greyson's hand, I kept having horrible thoughts. *What if she steps on a piece of glass while Greyson is running right behind her? Ugh. Why does my brain keep doing this?* I kept thinking of all the different ways Greyson or I could get infected. *Stop, stop, stop thinking about it,* I berated myself. Remember, it was 1996, and HIV was a taboo subject. There were a lot of unknowns to the general public.

Well, of course, Anna never stepped on a piece of glass, and I'm sure the scrape on her hand was minuscule or she would've been like, "I'm bleeding." Duh. So looking back, I was not being rational. I just couldn't relax around Anna anymore. I was eager to get back to Oklahoma (said no one ever). If we had cell phones back then, I would've called 1-800-AID-AIDS eighty-two times during my twelve-hour drive home in search of a better answer regarding my mosquito bites. I was young . . . and uninformed . . . and sad —really, really sad . . . with a dash of crazy.

MATTHEW 7:1–5

1997–1998

*A*nna was in full swing working in Los Angeles again. She was working on a movie with George Clooney. She never spoke much about work or the stars she worked with, but she did talk about George. George said this, and George said that. George did this, and George did that. I'd never heard her smitten with anyone. Not even William. Anna wasn't the smitten type. She was the I-don't-have-time-for-men-because-all-I-do-is-work type. Clearly, she knew George Clooney was out of reach considering she had AIDS and, well, he's George Clooney. But she did form a bit of a friendship with him. Anna told me about their conversations and all the hilarious things he did. She said she'd never met a man like him before. She said he was so nice to everyone on set and not pretentious at all. When she was offered a small role on his next film, *Three Kings*, she was ecstatic.

I also had a new job. I'd gotten a teaching position at a Baptist preschool three days a week. That was another perfect job for me because Greyson was able to come with me and attend preschool for free. I taught the four-year-olds, so Greyson wasn't in my class, which was a good thing. Like most children, Greyson behaved better for strangers. I prayed he wouldn't have episodes at school.

A couple months went by and work was going well. The parents and students seemed happy to have me as a teacher. My boss liked me and gave me positive feedback about everything I was doing in the classroom. Greyson was doing okay, but I often wondered if his sweet teachers would give me bad news. Greyson's class seemed to have the winning formula—two teachers, only ten students, a giant classroom full of books and toys, and an outdoor area to run free.

I did make a mistake of popping my head in once to say hi, and Greyson had an episode. Imagine the scene from the movie *Alien* where the alien tries to get Sigourney Weaver. It was like that. His teachers restrained him while his body and arms flapped about uncontrollably. I quickly left the scene but noticed one of the teachers pulling him into the supply room next door. It seemed that my popping in but not taking him threw him off. He didn't understand that the school day wasn't over yet. *Mental note to self: Never say hi to Greyson at school.*

The more I thought about it, the more I wondered how the teachers acted so quickly and seemed to know how to handle Greyson's episode. When I approached his teachers after school, they said it had only happened a couple of times. Who am I not to believe two Christian women with wide eyes, squeaky voices, and smiles that show every tooth?

Since I only worked three days a week, the other four days Greyson and I did everything together. We were inseparable. Greyson was difficult, but he also made life interesting because he was unlike anyone else. Greyson encompassed the meaning of "God broke the mold when He made you." I had never loved anyone so much in my life. I never even knew I was capable of such love. My parents were crazy in love with Greyson too. My dad read to Greyson every single night. And not just one or two books—he read to Greyson for an hour every night. I read to Greyson every night too. Greyson could sit and listen to books for hours on end. He had an unusually long attention span. I would describe Greyson's attention span as a constant state of "hyperfocusivity"—(yeah, I just made up another word there)—particularly with things like puzzles, books, or anything Batman–related.

When Greyson was three, he went through a stage where he'd only wear his Batman costume. Luckily, it was a pretty simplistic costume, but it did have a cape. I learned with Greyson that I had to pick my battles, so after beginning several days with a forty-five minute beating, I decided that was no longer a battle I wanted to fight. Greyson wore his Batman costume every day for months. He even wore it to school. Fortunately, his teachers supported me since they'd witnessed what Greyson was capable of a few times. I guess Greyson rubbed off on the rest of the class because I often saw a Superman and Robin show up too. I'm sure his teachers loved having a room full of students who could leap tall buildings in a single bound.

My parents continued to buy Greyson and me passes to the zoo and science museum, so we went several times a month. Also, from the time he was about a year old, I took him to live performances. He was probably the only one-year-old to sit through *Sesame Street Live!* without moving a muscle. Greyson and I also frequented the local playgrounds, water parks, and indoor play centers. My parents were so generous funding our entertainment because they wanted to make sure Greyson had a very happy and fun childhood. We could never tell by Greyson's face that he was having fun since he never smiled or laughed or showed emotion, but he must've been having fun at all those great places, right?

By that time, I hadn't dated for almost four years, which was really a shame since I looked so damn good. I peaked physically just in time for men to run because I had a child. It was like God was playing a prank on me. He's such a silly fella.

I craved a relationship with a good man—not a Michael, a good man. That was one reason why I became so active in the born-again Christian community. I thought where better to meet a good man than at church? And I loved, loved, loved my church.

By then, I was used to the whole Friday night service thing. It's not like I had anything else going on Friday nights. I stopped going to my Catholic church, except occasionally with my parents, but I never missed a Friday night at my nondenominational church full of born-again Christians. It really was the highlight of my week. The service was actually fun: the pastor was really engaging and the music was pretty decent. But even though I attended that amazing church every Friday night, never once did a man approach me. I had to drop off Greyson at the church preschool right before the service and pick him up right after, so everyone could see I had a son. I often felt men looking at me, but it was all over when they saw Greyson. Every week, I made sure I hung out a little while after the service, pretending to be interested in the pictures on the wall, just praying someone would talk to me, but it never happened. Not one man—or woman for that matter—approached me in over two years at that church. Every week, I sat alone. Friendless. It actually felt like I was being shunned, but of course, that's not possible in a church. Is it?

I was also an active participant in multiple Bible study groups during those couple years. Men often spoke to me during Bible study, but as soon as I mentioned Greyson, they were like, buh-bye. I could sense when men found me attractive, but I also felt the lights go out simultaneously when I mentioned that I had a son. I thought Christians weren't supposed to be judgmental, but I began to wonder if that was true.

I eventually joined a Christian singles group that met weekly. I was excited because there was no connection between my church, my Bible study groups, or this singles group, so no one knew me. When I showed up for my first meeting, I was pleasantly surprised that the group was enormous. There were about 200 single men and women. I strategically sat at a table with attractive men and was pleased with the amount of attention I received. I decided to keep Greyson out of my conversations just for shits and giggles, and by the end of the night, I'd been invited to a party.

All this newfound attention called for a little experiment.

When I arrived at the party, I noticed that only the attractive people from the singles group were there, so I guess I made the cut. I took a particular liking to a guy named Brad. He was really charismatic and cute. Brad seemed to take quite an interest in me as well. I was also getting along with several other men in the group, and the women seemed to like me as well. I started to feel excited for the first time in years. I left the party feeling rejuvenated.

The next week I went to the singles group again, and again I was invited to a party—a barbecue. I was beginning to feel like a social life was actually possible. It had been so long that I'd forgotten what it was like hanging out with people my own age. Other than seeing Rachel and Anna in Chicago every summer for a couple weeks, social interactions with friends had been nonexistent.

I showed up at the cute-Christians-only barbecue and was my usual charming self. Brad gave me extra attention as did a couple of the other guys. It was like my options went from zero to ten in two weeks. Brad invited me to a dinner party the group was having the following weekend. I told him I'd be there and his interest in me was palpable. I had not been on a date in four years, but I wasn't stupid. Not anymore.

My experiment of not mentioning Greyson wasn't difficult to manage because the subject of children never came up in a group of single churchgoers—especially during our weekly meetings at the church because those meetings were very structured around biblical teachings and only allowed for limited mingling. But now that I had attended two parties and was invited to a third by yummy Brad, I started teetering between being okay with my experiment and feeling deceptive now that friendships were forming. So I decided to come clean.

I waited for a seamless moment to weasel Greyson into the conversation so it seemed natural and unplanned.

There. I did it. I said Greyson's name. Casually.

"Oh, so you have a son?" A guest responded in a pretend-to-be-interested, high-pitched voice.

"Yes, he's three," I said, mustering up my greatest fake smile. I instantaneously felt the energy in the room shift.

There went my social life. It was as if I'd announced I had the plague. As word of my son spread throughout the intimate barbecue, the men dropped like flies. Conversations with women and attention from men shifted away from me instead of toward me. Soon thereafter, I saw my way out of the barbecue and drove home, tears rolling down my face.

I decided to go to the weekly meeting at the Christian singles group one more time, just in case I'd hallucinated all my newfound friends and love interests rejecting me, instead of supporting me, because I was a single mom. Not one single person who showed an interest in me at the first party or the barbecue ever spoke to me again. Not one single word.

And the dinner party I was invited to by Brad was never mentioned again, so needless to say, I was uninvited. It was disappointing that the women ostracized me as well. It was like they didn't want to be friends with the woman who had sinned.

I found it confusing—or maybe hypocritical is a better word—that southern born-again Christians seemed to preach one thing but do the exact opposite. I'd never been treated more like an outcast than I was in the born-again Christian community. All the church services and Bible study groups I'd attended over the years discussed things like not passing judgment, accepting and loving one another, being kind and compassionate to others, encouraging one another, and being sympathetic. But as I examined the obvious shift in how I'd been treated since becoming a single mother in a southern state full of born-again Christians, I began to realize that born-again Christians were perhaps the most judgmental, intolerant, discouraging, and merciless people I had ever known. *Maybe it's just an Oklahoma thing?* I wondered.

On a side note, fast-forward a couple years. That's when I found out that the beloved, charismatic, and engaging pastor at the born-again Christian church I'd attended ran off with the church secretary, leaving his wife and three children behind. Can I get an Amen?

BACK TO THE MIDWEST

1998

I couldn't handle Oklahoma and all its hypocritical born-again Christians another day. I actively tried for three solid years to fit in with them and never made a single friend among their ranks. In the past, my personality was to blame, but not anymore. By that point in my life, I'd become friggin' lovely. Southern born-again Christians just couldn't accept me and the fact that I was a single mom. They must've figured they were just way too good for a slut like me. Apparently, all born-again Christians have never had sex. But I'd bet big bucks that I'd had way less sex in my life than most of the people in that Christian singles group of 200 people. I'd even bet a couple of those women had had abortions. But Jesus forgave them. Apparently, it doesn't count if people don't find out.

I had to get out of Oklahoma and move back to the Midwest, but I didn't have any family in Chicago anymore except my sister who I knew would never help me with Greyson. At that point, Alice was thirty-seven years old and had absolutely no interest in having children, being around children, or interacting with children in any way, shape, or form. So I decided to move to Minnesota near the only other family I had in the Midwest. I had an aunt, uncle, and three cousins who lived near Minneapolis. It was difficult and, looking back, incredibly stupid to leave my parents, but I needed my independence, and more importantly, I needed out of Oklahoma. So I did it. Like ripping off a Band-Aid, I just packed up our stuff and drove to Minnesota. *Next best thing to Chicago here I come!*

My aunt and uncle were so kind to take Greyson and me into their home while I got on my feet. I started looking for a teaching job the day after I arrived and was hired within two weeks as a full-time preschool teacher at a Catholic school. Then I immediately found an apartment, and three weeks after arriving in Minnesota, I moved out of my aunt and uncle's home.

My new apartment was great. It had an electric fireplace, which I didn't even know was a thing. I just flipped a switch, and voilà, fire! It heated up the whole modest-sized apartment, which was a huge plus in Minnesota. I loved the apartment but could only afford a one bedroom with my $18,000 salary. I gave Greyson the bedroom and just pretended the living room was a studio apartment. I didn't have any furniture, and I couldn't afford actual beds, so I bought a twin mattress for Greyson and a full-sized mattress for me. I just put Greyson's mattress on the floor in his room and my mattress on the floor in the living room. I bought a plastic dresser for each of us. It didn't bother me that we slept on mattresses on the floor. We were both perfectly comfortable and enjoyed living there very much.

I really liked my new job too. I shared teaching responsibilities with another teacher named Natalie. We were both certified teachers with equal say and responsibility. We shared four preschool programs—two morning and two afternoon classes. We had three-year-olds on Tuesdays and Thursdays and four-year-olds on Mondays, Wednesdays, and Fridays.

I enrolled Greyson in my afternoon class on Mondays, Wednesdays, Fridays. The rest of the time, he went to the school's day care center, which was an all-day program located down the hallway. I was nervous about Greyson being in my class, but every child in the day care attended one of the four preschool programs.

Even though Greyson was enrolled in two different programs, he had an established routine right from the start, so he did okay-ish. But he still had occasional episodes at school. A few times he had to be restrained by his day care teachers and by Natalie and me, but for the most part, his behavior during school hours was somewhat acceptable. It is typical, even for the average child, to behave better at school than at home.

However, a few months into the school year, Greyson's episodes got much worse after he befriended a boy named Cody. And by befriended, I mean that Greyson became obsessed with Cody, and Cody was like, "Greyson who?" Both Cody and Greyson were in my afternoon class of four-year-olds. So every Monday, Wednesday, and Friday after school, Greyson had an episode when Cody's mom picked him up to take him home. Greyson would hang onto Cody, refuse to let go, and scream until he was sweaty and red in the face. When I tried to peel Greyson off Cody, Greyson would hit me uncontrollably, and I would have to restrain him for the usual forty-five minutes. Natalie would finish up our work while I restrained Greyson, which obviously was not a good situation. Luckily, Cody's mom and I had already formed a friendly parent-teacher relationship before Greyson started displaying these behaviors. She was very happy with Natalie and me as Cody's teachers, so she was very understanding and sweet about everything. She started taking Greyson home with her at pickup time so I could finish up my work in peace. Told you Catholics are cool.

Once my new life in Minnesota settled into a routine, I went looking for another church. Now that I was in the Midwest, I assumed Christians would be much more down-to-earth and less judgy. I wanted to find a large church to get involved in, finally make some friends, and possibly even meet a nice Christian man. A real one. Not the pretend kind. My aunt recommended a Baptist church, so I decided to check it out.

I attended a Sunday morning service that was mediocre and monotonous at best. It was old-school like all the Catholic churches I'd been to throughout my life. I did, however, perk up at the end of the service when they talked about their much-anticipated spin-off church that was opening soon. The pastor said it was going to be a singles church. As in a church for single people. Back in Oklahoma, I had belonged to that one singles group and multiple Bible study groups that predominantly consisted of single people, but I'd never heard of an entire church just for single people. I felt like I'd won the lottery.

I continued going to that church every Sunday for months, not because I loved it the way I loved my church in Muskogee, but because I was anxiously awaiting the new singles church anomaly. Every Sunday at the end of the service, the pastor gave updates as everyone, particularly me, counted down the projected opening of the new church. The new church sounded like it was going to be amazing. Services on Friday nights, Christian rock bands, endless social activities each month, and it was called The Rock. I loved that. I felt like I needed a rock in my life—an anchor and a sense of solidity and strength. I hadn't been that excited in a really long time. *A whole church full of women and men my age? Certainly I'll make friends there.* Plus, my aunt, uncle, and cousins were totally willing to take Greyson a few times a month, so I couldn't wait to start having a real social life for the first time in five years. I got that hopeful feeling again. That feeling I got when I went to those two parties in Muskogee. *This time things would be different.*

As I waited patiently for the big day to arrive, Greyson and I enjoyed exploring all the kid-friendly things to do in Minnesota. I was overly conscientious about spending quality time with Greyson and going to exciting, fun-filled places. Often Greyson wanted to go sledding or play in the snow, which may actually be the most painful pastime in existence, but I always did it because I knew he loved it and it made him happy. Well, I assumed it made him happy. I couldn't rely on typical social cues like smiling, but he asked to play in the snow, so that was a good indicator. He also sometimes had an episode when it was time to stop sledding due to this thing called nighttime. Greyson insisted that sledding in the pitch dark was perfectly safe, and there was no rational reason to stop. In his mind, what he wanted was the best and only option.

In the past when Greyson would have an episode, it used to concern me, but I was so hopeful—no, I was convinced—that he'd get better, that he'd outgrow those behaviors. But instead, at age four, his episodes started to petrify me.

He displayed what felt like an unwavering determination to hurt me.

Smack, smack, smack, smack!

He was faster now so his flailing arms were more difficult to catch.

Smack, smack, smack!

Panting with determination, his face would get red with anger and drenched in sweat.

Smack, smack!

His eyes appeared glazed over like a demon had sucked out his soul.

SMACK!

Then I'd hold his arms and hold his arms and hold his arms. And I'd tell him everything would be okay. But it didn't matter what I told him because his face was completely blank and expressionless—like Greyson had checked out and left the building.

Then, forty-five exhausting minutes later, the Greyson I loved and adored would return. And I'd tell myself not to be scared.

I would say about 99 percent of me listened, but that tiny 1 percent of me started to fear Greyson. That 1 percent started closing his bedroom door when I went to bed at night. Soon thereafter, that 1 percent attached bells to his doorknob so I could hear if the door moved in the middle of the night. Eventually, that 1 percent hid all the knives in the kitchen. I'd lie in bed and envision Greyson with a menacing look on his face getting a knife in the middle of the night and stabbing me a hundred times with his arms flailing about.

When Greyson was just four years old, that 1 percent of me wondered if he was schizophrenic.

THE ROCK

1999

fter months of anticipation, the grand opening of The Rock finally arrived. I was so excited I changed outfits five times while dancing around my apartment to No Doubt. Christian rock belonged in the church, not in my apartment.

I showed up with Greyson that grand opening Friday night, and it was just as I imagined it would be: hundreds of people my age in attendance, Christian rock playing in the background, and excitement in the air. Since it was a singles church, there was no childcare, but assuming that, I'd brought several books for Greyson to hyperfocus on during the service. I grabbed seats for us and enjoyed a captivating service full of great music, great energy, and a great sermon. I loved it almost as much as I did the church in Muskogee. Greyson was perfectly behaved thanks to his ability to be completely unaware of his surroundings when his nose was in a book. The night couldn't have gone better, and I left The Rock envisioning all the wonderful things in store for me there.

The next morning I woke up with a smile on my face.

Greyson and I were getting ready to head to the Minnesota Children's Museum when my phone rang.

"Hello."

"Hi, this is Pastor Matt from The Rock. Do you have a moment?"

"Oh hi! Yes. I loved the service last night!"

"I'm actually calling to talk to you about last night. I saw that you have a son, and I want to let you know that our home church would be a better fit for you and your son. The Rock is a singles church."

"But I am single." *You silly goose.*

"Yes, but here at The Rock, we feel our home Baptist church would be best for you and your son."

"Are you telling me I can't attend your church?" *Lemme go clean my ears.*

"Yes, that is what I called to tell you."

Are you from Oklahoma?

I started crying and spewing Bible verses that went against what he told me, but he continued to solemnly repeat that The Rock was not a place for my son and me.

That marked the day I stopped actively going to church.

For four solid years, I'd tenaciously tried and tried and tried to find my place in a Christian church, make Christian friends, and feel like I belonged somewhere. Born-again Christians are the nastiest group of people I have ever known in my life. I thought the cruel ones all congregated in the South. I was never treated differently for being the only white person at an African American college in Chicago before I had Greyson. I was never treated differently when I was the only straight person at my job when living in LA. I'd never felt discrimination in my life until I entered the world of born-again "Christians," which I have put in air quotes because they're so far removed from what Christians are supposed to be. They should call themselves born-again assholes—no quotes necessary.

This realization did not, however, impact my relationship with God or my Christian faith. I felt God was looking down at all those supposed born-again "Christians" and He too was saddened by the way they treated people. I continued to pray every night. I didn't need a church to have a relationship with God.

My job as a Catholic preschool teacher continued, and I really enjoyed teaching with Natalie. We created really unusual, educational centers for our students. Greyson's all-time favorite center was when Natalie and I collected old tools and electronics from the parents. We received a ton of donations and were able to make an elaborate workshop center. Students were able to take apart (and attempt to reassemble) typewriters, radios, blenders, toasters, et cetera, using real tools. Only four students were allowed in the center at a time, and it required close supervision—particularly when Greyson was there. That's all I needed for Greyson to take a hammer to someone's head or a screwdriver to an eye. Let's just say I "helped in the workshop" when Greyson was there. It was such a popular center that just like my after-school art program back in Muskogee, we had a daily sign-up sheet. Greyson signed up every time he came to class. He sometimes had an episode if he couldn't have a turn that day or when it was time to leave the workshop. *I should add appliances to the list of things Greyson could hyperfocus on.*

Another center we created, despite my horror, was a spider tree center. We had a small potted tree that Natalie set in the middle of a kiddie pool full of water. I remember her saying something about how spiders won't cross water or something like that, but all I heard was "spider tree." Natalie went outside daily and caught spiders to put on the tree. She also encouraged students to go on "spider hunts" so she could add their findings to our tree. When the students showed me their spiders, I sent them directly to Natalie. They weren't paying me enough to deal with spiders. Eventually, the tree became encased with spiderwebs created by spiders that supposedly stayed put because of the water. I have to admit it was pretty cool, but I never went within ten feet of that spider tree.

Being at a Catholic school, we had a "Jonah and the Whale" theme one week. Natalie and I turned a huge storage closet into what looked like the inside of a whale. We covered the entire inside of the closet with large, black garbage bags and taped "bones" made out of white construction paper to the plastic bags. Natalie brought in a black light to make the bones glow in the dark, and I brought in cans of tuna and put one in each corner to make the inside of the whale smell fishy. Then we took turns leading small groups of students inside the whale where we read the story of "Jonah and the Whale" to them. That was my all-time favorite center.

My school was located on a small hill that was perfect for preschoolers to go sledding during the seemingly endless Minnesota winters. During the winter months—which lasted approximately forever—students were allowed to bring their sleds every Thursday and Friday, and we would go sledding with them at recess.

We also had several field trips during the year. Natalie taught me how to turn an ordinary field trip into an extraordinary one. Once we had a field trip to the grocery store. Snore. Each student was given a short shopping list of produce to pick out to take home, so that was fun. When we went to the butcher section, the kids were full of questions. The students took an interest in the cow tongues for sale, so Natalie decided to purchase one. *What? Why? Gross!* The next day, we cooked it, and each student got a sample if they wanted to try it. I was surprised that almost every student wanted to try cow tongue. Thankfully, it's easy to fool preschoolers and make them believe you eat something when you really don't because I certainly wasn't going to try it. Then we voted whether we liked it, thought it was okay, or didn't like it, and graphed the results. The majority liked it. Who knew?

Natalie even learned a few things from me that year. I came up with some great art projects, and I also taught the students to dance. We had impromptu dance parties during class, and I also choreographed a little dance show. It was super-duper cute, and parents were invited to watch after school one day. One of the dances was to the song "YMCA," and, as you can imagine, three- and four-year-olds doing the YMCA dance was freaking hilarious, slash adorable. The parents laughed and cried happy tears during the whopping ten-minute show. Natalie was the dance-art type as much as I was the spider-tree-cow-tongue-eating type, so together we made a great team.

I could fill this whole book with all the great things we did that year. Natalie taught me how to make learning interesting, fun, and thought-provoking. She taught me to modify instruction based on student interest and direction instead of based on what I wrote in my lesson plan book. She taught me that when I set my expectations high, my students would surprise me. I also learned that teaching isn't about instruction, it's about encouraging exploration so students can find answers on their own.

Unfortunately, I only had one year at that school. Even though I was well-liked by my principal and I loved my job, there was one thing about Minnesota I couldn't stand. It snowed. A lot. I mean a lot, a lot. On our last day of school in June, we had plans to have a picnic at a nearby lake. But in

Minnesota, a June picnic can get snowed out. Snow from early October to June was something even my Chicago blood couldn't handle. People who voluntarily chose to live in Minnesota made no sense to me.

PS—Even with all of Greyson's episodes, I never felt judged at that Catholic school. Not from Natalie, not from my principal who was a nun, not from the other teachers, and not from my students' parents. I loved my first year as a classroom teacher at that wonderful Catholic school.

Peace out Minnesota.

QUEEN LINDA

1999

*R*ealizing I didn't want to live in Antarctica came at a good time. My mother had just retired from teaching, and my parents bought a home in California about an hour away from where my brother lived in San Diego. My father had another year until he could retire, but my mom was eager to begin life as a retired woman in sunny California and decorate their new home. I told her I would go to California with her and help her get settled until Dad could join her. Sunny California sounded pretty good after experiencing snow in June. My father had enough frequent flyer miles to fly around the universe, so he was able to visit all the time.

So off I went to California with my mom and Greyson. When we arrived, the sunshine, warm breeze, and palm trees reminded me of Anna and all the great times we'd had living in Los Angeles. I didn't get that feeling of home like I did in Chicago, but it was definitely an upgrade from Minnesota.

I immediately went looking for a teaching job, but since I had an out-of-state license, I had to stick with a private school again. There weren't any Catholic schools in the small town we moved to in Southern California, but there was a Christian school. *Meh. A Christian school doesn't necessarily mean a born-again Christian school, does it?* I was desperate, so I applied.

After two interviews at the Christian school, I landed a first grade teaching position. I felt like "The Shit" because I found out that the school was quite prestigious. Back then, in 1999, the tuition for one year at the school was equivalent to the cost of my entire college degree. Plus, Greyson could attend the school for free, so that was a bonus.

I was hoping Greyson's episodes would subside once he was a big kindergartner. But before he could be accepted into the school's program, he had to be tested. Apparently, subpar children weren't allowed. After Greyson finished his tests, they came out of the room and looked at me like they'd just seen Jesus. "You have one very smart cookie," they said.

My new principal was scary as fuck and was nothing like the sweet little nun I'd worked for in Minnesota. The skin on her face was very taut, and she wore her makeup too perfectly. She also used much too much hairspray on her sculpted hair. Sometimes, I wanted to light a cigarette to see if her head would blow up. She wore impeccably tailored suits, the kind with pleats. I think she stood in her office all day because she never had a wrinkle in a suit—or her taut skin. Every suit was accessorized with a brooch. I've never worn a brooch or a suit for that matter. I've never understood brooches. Why put a pin through an $800 suit? And her name was Linda. I don't like Lindas.

I went into work a week before school started to set up my classroom. While working, Linda summoned me into her office. Her office looked nothing like the sister's quaint little office in Minnesota. Linda's office had a professional desk with decorative trim, beautiful pictures hanging on the walls, lavish window treatments, and built-in shelves adorned with worldly trinkets showcasing her travels. I couldn't help thinking, *I don't think I'm getting paid enough.*

Linda offered me a piece of gold-wrapped chocolate. *Gold-wrapped? The platinum-wrapped chocolates must be on back order.* I grabbed a piece and threw it in my purse. I'm not one to turn down substandard chocolate.

Linda took our one-on-one opportunity to tell me what was expected of me that year. She spoke very methodically, like a politician. No, more like a queen. She enunciated every word just perfectly. "If you leave before five, you must carry a full tote of work to complete at home. You must have a new theme in your classroom every two weeks. The theme shall be represented in your lesson plans, bulletin boards, and displayed artwork. All lesson plans must include an objective, introduction, step-by-step instructions, assessment tool, closing, and state standards. Weekly lesson plans must be in my mailbox every Monday morning by eight. Every word exchanged with parents must be documented—all conferences, phone calls, even conversations at arrival and dismissal. Everything. Anything shy of these expectations shall result in coming in on Saturday. Not Sunday. Sunday is for worshipping our Lord."

"Oooo-kaaaay," I said, looking puzzled. "Absolutely!" I added with a mustered-up fake smile and a side of fake enthusiasm. *No problem, Queen Linda. But I'm most definitely not getting paid enough.* People always assume private school teachers get paid more than public school teachers, but private school teachers get paid significantly less.

I returned to my room in a state of what-the-hell-just-happened. My principal was actually more frightening than she looked. I popped that gold-wrapped chocolate in my mouth hoping for a liquor-filled center. *Damn this chocolate is delicious. I should've grabbed two.* I then proceeded to turn my classroom into what looked like a magical wonderland. *My principal may be scary, but I enjoy a challenge.*

At the beginning of the school year, I got Greyson into therapy hoping it would lessen his episodes. At this point, he was five years old, and in 1999, this was supposedly the age autism could be diagnosed. I was anxious to hear what the therapist had to say. Up until then, every time I mentioned Greyson's behaviors to a doctor, they'd say, "he's fine" or "he's in a phase."

Greyson's therapist, Dr. Patel, was kind and very calm. During our first appointment, he asked me a lot of questions and took a lot of notes. He spent the next few appointments interacting with Greyson and observing his behavior. Within a month, Dr. Patel reported three diagnoses: First, there was sensory integration—now known as sensory processing disorder (SPD), a condition in which the brain has difficulty managing information received through the senses. Greyson's SPD caused him to have an oversensitivity to things in his environment that he considered bothersome, such as tags in clothing, textures of foods, and seeing things out of place. However, his severely heightened SPD challenges were in the social, emotional, and self-regulating areas, which caused his inability to get along, interact reciprocally, and make connections with others.

Next, there was oppositional defiant disorder (ODD)—a mental health disorder that causes frequent and persistent irritability, anger, vindictiveness, defiance, and argumentative behavior. Greyson's ODD was exhibited through his difficulty to get along with others, explosive outbursts, and abusive behavior. Behaviors relating to ODD often intensify in the home where the child feels more safe, but they can also extend to other settings. That explained why Greyson was sometimes okay in church, at school, or outside the home with me.

Finally, Dr. Patel diagnosed Greyson with autism, which now falls under the umbrella of autism spectrum disorder (ASD) due to the vast range of symptoms. ASD is a developmental disorder that causes differences in the brain resulting in difficulties with communication, social interaction, and behavior. Avoiding eye contact, obsessive interests, sleep problems, and an inability to express enjoyment were some of the characteristics Greyson exhibited. Dr. Patel did note, however, that Greyson didn't fit the autism mold. He wasn't mute, didn't rock, and had no developmental delays—characteristics predominantly used to diagnose autism in 1999. Greyson also handled an abundance of preferable stimuli well, particularly environments that exercised his brain—like the museum, theater, or zoo—which is not typical of people with autism or SPD.

Dr. Patel seemed perplexed and a little unsure of his autism diagnosis. He said he'd never met another child like Greyson. Like everyone who spent time with Greyson, Dr. Patel was astonished by his intelligence. He agreed with me that Greyson was extraordinary. *Finally! Someone else sees it!*

School began and my students were lovely. The parents were kind and seemed very happy with me. Maybe a little too happy, though, because they loved chatting with me. Which was great and all, except that I had to document every word. Every time Queen Linda caught me chatting with a parent, she'd later pull me aside and ask if I'd documented the conversation.

"I just asked if they enjoyed their camping trip."

"Document it."

"What they told me about their camping trip?" I may have accidentally looked at her like she was insane.

"Yes, document it, please. I'd also like to check all your documentation thus far, so please make a copy of all your notes and put them in my mailbox. Thank you."

Queen Linda needs to get laid.

I wasn't sure how the other teachers did it. I was staying at work every day until six to free me from a work-filled tote. Plus, I worked every single Saturday, all day long. It seemed that as soon as I got all the students' artwork displayed and the bulletin boards revamped, it was time to change them again. Before the school year began, it took me a whole week to make my room beautiful *without* students, how was I supposed to do a full makeover in my room every two weeks when I was teaching all day long? Once I kept a theme for three weeks to see if Queen Linda would notice. She did. She vocalized her displeasure, and I stayed at work until nine o'clock that night. I couldn't wait to hear about her displeasure with my notes.

Queen Linda liked to pop into my classroom unannounced about once a week. She always stayed for around thirty minutes then left me a note on monogrammed stationery. She sure loved notes. Much to my surprise, she always wrote what a great job I did teaching. *Surely she can think of something patronizing to write.*

Copies of my beyond-detailed lesson plans were in Queen Linda's mailbox every Monday morning by eight o'clock sharp. She would return the copies with little handwritten comments like "Assessment tool?" and highlight it. I began triple-checking my lesson plans each week to avoid her little highlighted comments. Little did she know that I typically did my lesson plans Sunday morning, which interfered with my worshipping-the-Lord time.

In addition to having to deal with Queen Linda, Greyson's kindergarten teacher was extremely impersonal. She hardly ever said a word to me, which I thought was strange since we were colleagues. But then I realized that even though we were colleagues, I was also the parent of one of her students, so she was probably trying to avoid documenting every word. *Smart. I should try to say fewer words.* I assumed no news was good news regarding Greyson, so maybe therapy was working.

By a couple months into the school year, I was full of mom guilt because I was constantly working and Greyson wasn't accustomed to spending so little time with me. In Minnesota, Natalie and I left every day by four thirty and I never worked on weekends, yet we still managed to do an amazing job. Queen Linda's expectations were so unreasonable that my time with Greyson was limited to dinner, reading at night, and something fun every Sunday after I finished my lesson plans.

Luckily, my mom picked up the slack and spent a lot of time with Greyson. For some reason, he rarely attacked her. I figured it was because she had a bad case of grandmaitis—a condition many grandmothers have that often results in the inability to say no and the severe spoiling of grandchildren. She and my dad were the only other people who knew of Greyson's diagnoses, so together we took that pertinent information and tackled Greyson's challenges head-on. Just joshing—we completely ignored it, fully believing our love and Greyson's intelligence would conquer all.

Sometimes I wondered if my parents ever felt afraid of Greyson, but I would never ask because I'd have to say those words out loud. (Plus, I already knew their answer would be, "Of course not!") Looking back, I realize that my denial, internalization of feelings, and dedication to politeness attributed to my excruciating loneliness. I had so much weighing on me, but I never confided in a single soul.

Halloween and Thanksgiving had come and gone, and the teaching aspect of my job was going great. I really loved teaching and my students, but the long hours were wearing on me. I tried one more time to get away with a three-week theme before redecorating my entire classroom, but nothing got past Queen Linda. She wasn't too thrilled with my notes either—even though every day after school I spent twenty to thirty minutes documenting conversations. She knew I spoke with parents much more than I documented, and she was right. I picked two parents to call each week just to tell them what a great job their child was doing, and I definitely never documented that. If Queen Linda got word, she would've started looking for those conversations in my notes too.

Around the first week of December, the drama teacher frantically burst into my classroom and said that Linda needed me in her office immediately. The drama teacher stayed with my students while I ran out of the room.

When I arrived at Queen Linda's office, Greyson was there in the middle of an episode. Her office was in total disarray—papers covered the ground, her chair was knocked over, and her worldly knickknacks were scattered about.

Uh-oh.

Queen Linda was sitting on the floor in her $800 suit trying to restrain Greyson. Spit flew from his mouth as he screamed. Sweat dripped down his red face. His blank eyes never acknowledged my presence. The veins in his neck bulged as his little body violently wriggled to escape her tight grip. Queen Linda desperately hid her face to avoid getting hurt.

When she looked up, our eyes locked. Her teeth were

clenched, her eyes were squinted, her face was clammy, and her perfectly coiffed hair was a mess. Her nose was dripping, but not with blood like mine had a few times in the past during Greyson's episodes.

As I took over the Greyson-restraining duties and got smacked several times, I noticed a chunk of Queen Linda's hair in his fist. Queen Linda angrily wiped her nose with her sleeve then desperately stroked her clothes with her hands in an unsuccessful attempt to regain her composure. *There's that wrinkle in her suit I've been looking for.*

Livid, she articulated how Greyson hit her repeatedly then proceeded to list all the items Greyson threw at her. I was mortified to hear that one of the items was her chair. Okay, maybe 99 percent mortified, 1 percent satisfied.

Queen Linda then stormed out of her office looking disheveled for the first time in her life. As I continued to restrain Greyson, I maneuvered my position so one hand could quickly grab all the gold-wrapped chocolates scattered within reach on the floor. I used my teeth to open one, then tossed it in my mouth. Slumped on the floor, I numbly held my uncontrollable son, sucked on a creamy chocolate with a delightfully crunchy exterior, stared at a crooked picture on the wall, and wondered, *Why?*

Thirty minutes and six chocolates later, Greyson settled down. His episodes still lasted about forty-five minutes each time.

Queen Linda reemerged as I was painstakingly trying to replicate her knickknack arrangement. Greyson was quietly sitting on her now upright chair like nothing had ever happened. He was reading a book I found on the floor.

Still heated, Queen Linda said, "Greyson has been out of control in class several times."

"That was never mentioned to me by his teacher."

"Perhaps his teacher thought she could handle it."

"Perhaps collaborating with his mom would've been helpful."

"Enroll Greyson somewhere else."

And that was that. Greyson's teacher not communicating with me gave me hope that he was doing better, but in reality, he was doing worse. Perhaps after working for Queen Linda a few years, his teacher got to a point where she simply no longer communicated with parents. On the one hand, I can't say that I blame her because it was such a note-taking time-saver. But the more I thought about the lack of communication from Greyson's teacher and Queen Linda, the more infuriated I became. I had been working my ass off trying my damnedest to meet Queen Linda's ridiculous expectations, but she didn't even have the decency to inform me of what was going on with Greyson. Where were *her* fucking notes?

A few days later I turned in my letter of resignation, which I'm pretty sure is status quo when your son tries to murder your boss. At that point, I'd hit rock bottom. I was a single mom of a five-year-old who was labeled with three diagnoses and had been kicked out of school. *What child gets kicked out of kindergarten?* I'd worked so hard to be a great teacher and now what? *Could I even put a half year on my résumé? "Reason for leaving: Son brutally attacked boss."* Not only that, but I hadn't been on a date in *six years!* I'd turned into a beautiful woman just to spend my life between a classroom and Chuck E. Cheese. I didn't even have any friends except Anna who was dying and Rachel who was in marital bliss. And I missed Chicago. Chicago reminded me of when life was good. I wanted my life to be good again.

I was so sad.

So very, very sad.

This was not what I'd envisioned for my life at age twenty-seven. Anna and I were supposed to be living it up in

Chicago and LA. I wanted to go back to the days when Anna and I passed 200 people in line, gave a hug to the bouncer, then got in the hip nightclubs for free. I wanted to go back to the days when men were vying for our attention and sending us drinks. I wanted to go back to the days of tiramisu-hopping and sitting in a dressing room drinking Slurpees. All I had was an autistic son who beat the shit out of me and got kicked out of kindergarten. *How did I get from that life to this life so quickly?*

I was friendless.

Manless.

Moneyless.

Jobless.

Sexless.

Funless.

I wrote a letter to my students' parents telling them I would not be returning after Christmas break, which I'm pretty sure came as no surprise since word had gotten around that Queen Linda had kicked my son out of school. I was so devastated because I had the most wonderful students and parents. I thought they'd be upset at me for leaving.

But it was quite the contrary—the reactions of my students and their parents were beautiful. I received countless letters of appreciation and support. Everyone understood my predicament. Parents showered me with Christmas presents—nice, expensive presents. But my favorite one was a gorgeous, handmade Christmas quilt. The mom wrote a sweet note in the corner with a Sharpie. She was the mom of my most-challenging student whom I adored. I still smile when I take out that quilt every year at Christmastime.

It was only a few months until my father would join my mom in California, so I told her I wanted to go back to Chicago after Christmas. She never told me no because all she wanted was for me to be happy. I'd been trying to return to Chicago for six years, and it felt like the right time. It was awful of me to leave her all alone in a new town. I was a crappy daughter during that time of depression and desperation, but that's what I did. I left my mom and went back to Chicago in search of my old life.

*I*t felt great to be in Chicago again. For the first time in over six years, I couldn't stop smiling, even though it was January and like a thousand degrees below zero. You must think I'm crazy for leaving Southern California for Chicago in the middle of winter, but that just shows how desperate I was to return to my beloved city. And at least it wouldn't be snowing in June like it did in Minnesota.

However, I didn't know anyone in Chicago anymore except Anna, Rachel, and my sister. Sadly, by that time, Anna was bedridden and getting progressively worse. She was never able to fulfill her small role in the movie *Three Kings* with George Clooney. When we spoke on the phone, she had difficulty holding a conversation. It was heart-wrenching to hear her knowing what a vibrant woman she once was. She got upset anytime I mentioned visiting her. She didn't want me to see her so weak and fragile. Anna had taken well-deserved pride in her strength, independence, and resilience her entire life, and now she could barely move or eat. I was in a constant state of anguish because she was always on my mind.

The only people left that I knew in Chicago were blissfully married Rachel and my sister, Alice. But Alice and I were no longer close like we were when I was little. She was living with her boyfriend, Ed, in his apartment, and he wasn't too happy when I asked if Greyson and I could stay with them while I looked for a job. Ed told me he'd give me two weeks and two weeks only.

I frantically applied for jobs everywhere, but there were no teaching jobs since it was January. My dad suggested I apply at a company in the area that had landed a spot on *Fortune* magazine's list of the 100 best places to work in America, so I did.

I quickly landed an interview there, and it went really well. They called me in for a second interview, and that went well too. They scheduled a third interview, but, by that time, my two-week welcome at the apartment was up. Ed would not extend my stay until I found out whether I'd gotten the job, so I had to find an apartment in, like, a day.

I took the first apartment that would take me without having a job. I had to pay three months' rent up front *and* a security deposit since I was jobless, but at least they took me. That ate up almost all my savings from my teaching job in California.

My third interview went great, and I got the job just days after Ed kicked Greyson and me out. Consequently, I ended up stuck in an apartment an hour away from my new job. However, Ed did sell me a sofa he no longer wanted for $600. What a guy! That gobbled up the rest of my savings, but I was happy to own a piece of furniture that wasn't made of plastic.

Before January was over, I enrolled Greyson in school and started my new job. I was hired in the marketing department as a media specialist, which is code for writer and editor. Technically, my position was intended for someone with a degree in marketing, but they liked that I had teaching experience and a degree in education. By this time, I was starting to realize that I'm really good at this interviewing stuff.

My salary was up to $30,000, so I could afford childcare. Kind of. My hours were eight to five, which was okay, I guess, except for the fact that I lived a fucking hour away. During my two-hour drive each day, I cursed Ed knowing that the dreaded commute could've been avoided if he'd just allowed Greyson and me to stay a few more days.

My boss's name was Janet, and she was an odd bird. She was only a couple years older than me, but she looked like an old frump. She didn't wear makeup and wore glasses from the '80s—or so they appeared—which didn't make sense since the company we worked for offered a vision benefit that paid for new glasses each year. So either she was really lazy or had really bad taste. I'm guessing bad taste because her hair was also feathered. *Who feathers their hair in the year 2000? Does she think she's Farrah Fawcett? I wish I could assure her that she's not.* She looked frumpy, dressed frumpy, and acted frumpy. She didn't like me, my long blonde hair, my supercute clothes, or my bubbly personality. She was a big, dull, frumpy grump. I missed my principal from Minnesota.

My first day on the job, I sat down with Erin, the woman assigned to train me. It was on my very first day that I realized something crucial: I didn't know how to type. Erin looked at me like, *You have got to be kidding me.* It's a good thing they never asked during my interviews if I could type. Although, I totally would've lied. I'd never had a computer before, so it never even crossed my mind. Teachers didn't have computers back then. All my lesson plans, newsletters, and wretched Queen Linda notes were all handwritten.

Luckily, I'd taken a typing class in high school and remembered the fundamentals like where to set my fingers. I'd earned a C in that class and really wished I would've paid more attention. Nevertheless, I taught myself how to type really well in less than two weeks. I'm pretty sure all the women in the department were rightfully giggling at me as I learned to type. They thought I was an airhead. I looked like an airhead. Let's just say it wasn't the best first impression I've ever made. But at least I had a job. Now I just needed a social life.

Rachel actually found time in her perfect life to invite me to a party. Yay! A party! I hadn't been to a non-born-again Christian party in over six years. I was supposed to be in the prime of my life, yet I never had any fun—except zoo, park, sledding, swimming, museum, Lego, Batman kind of fun. And we all know that's not really fun—unless you're five.

I got all decked out and showed up at the party. I felt a little awkward since I only knew Rachel and her husband. Then this guy named Sam started talking to me. An actual real male person started talking to me. We traded small talk all night, but I wasn't attracted to him. I talked about Greyson a bit, even though I'd been trained to think that being a mom was a man repellent. But I honestly didn't care if Sam was into me or not. I kept our conversation on the surface level. I wasn't like, "By the way, I have a son with autism, oppositional defiant disorder, and sensory processing disorder, who beats me up, got kicked out of kindergarten, and completely altered my career path." Yeah, it sounds really bad when I put it like that. True, but bad.

I was actually incredibly proud of Greyson. I loved him more than anything that ever existed in the world. I knew he was complicated. I knew he was difficult. I knew he was atypical. But looking back and knowing what I know now, I also knew he was going to be the next Steve Jobs or a real-life Sheldon Cooper: awkward yet wicked smart. That was how I envisioned future adult Greyson—except that 1 percent of me that feared him. In the very back of my brain, I tucked away the thought that Greyson was schizophrenic . . . or a serial killer. I kept that 1 percent to myself. Always. I loved him way too much for that to really be true.

The party was small and, truth be told, a little bit boring. I could only handle so much perfect Rachel and her perfect husband talking about their perfect life. And Sam certainly wasn't doing it for me, so I decided to head out. I was paying Rachel's niece to babysit, and I didn't think Sam was worth the five bucks an hour I was paying her. But when he followed me to my car and asked for my number, I thought, *Oh, what the hell. No one has asked for my number in over six years.* So I gave Sam my number.

Well of course Sam called me, since I really didn't want him to. He asked me out to dinner. I closed my eyes, squished up my face, pursed my lips, and muttered an unenthusiastic "Okay." But in my head, I was thinking, *I've got to hire a babysitter for this?*

Sam came to pick me up and took me to a nice steakhouse—the kind of steakhouse where everything was à la carte. That made it a little more worth my time. I hadn't been to a nice restaurant since I'd dated Sperm Donor. I hadn't been on a date since Sperm Donor. I wished I found Sam remotely desirable. *I guess I can't have my steak and eat it too.*

Our date went surprisingly well. Sam was a great conversationalist. He was also very successful. He owned his own office supply company. And he wasn't unattractive. I'd describe him as a fine-looking man. But his eyebrows were too bushy, and his hairline was too weird. When you looked at him from behind, you could see where he got his hair cut, then two inches below that, you could see his hair growing in. Like his barber didn't know where his hairline was, and Sam never checked the back of his head. At least he had hair. Really thick hair. Maybe that was part of it—he was just too damn hairy. Like a handsome gorilla. He also wasn't very tall. I'm five eight and he was maybe five ten at best. So, to me, he was short, . . . and he had small feet. Correction, he was like a handsome *baby* gorilla.

After an incredible totally-made-it-worth-it steak and hours of great conversation, Sam drove me home. I quickly said thank you and good night to avoid any human contact.

By this time, Greyson had been in school for a few weeks and his teacher had already contacted me. (I highly doubt that she had to document every word of our conversation like I did for Queen Linda. Maybe she just made a simple notation that a call was made regarding his behavior. Otherwise known as a normal expectation. I was dying to ask her, but I didn't.) She talked about how Greyson was brilliant but had difficulties socially and keeping his hands to himself. She said that day her students had to evacuate the room because Greyson had had an outburst. Apparently, in public school you can't restrain students like you can in private school. Instead, all other students are removed from the area.

Greyson was off to a rocky start in school, but things were going pretty well at my new job. It appeared that I was actually a pretty good writer. Who knew? My job was to write and edit content for products. After that, a graphic artist would design the pages and then they were sent off to the printer. Every employee with the same job title as me was told to strive for a 10 percent redo rate on their pages. That meant when a manager reviewed the hard copy from the printer, 90 percent of the pages were approved and only 10 percent had to be redone before the entire catalog was printed and sent out to customers. Since I always took my jobs way too seriously, I strived for a 0 percent redo rate on my pages and hit it. In other words, my catalogs were flawless. My pages never had to be redone unless there was a printing error or something major like that.

Despite the fact that I was a rock star at my job, Janet, aka Frumpy, continued to dislike me. Occasionally, I would have to ask her a question, so I'd go to her cubicle and sit in the chair right outside that might as well had a sign on it that said, "Sit here if you want to talk to Frumpy." But when I sat in that chair, Frumpy ignored me. She knew I was sitting there. And she knew that I knew that she knew I was sitting there. She had a wide-open, half-walled cubicle, and the chair sat within the boundaries of her direct vision. But Frumpy would just keep typing and typing like she was so incredibly busy that she didn't have five minutes to spare. She'd eventually sigh, and say with as little enthusiasm as humanly possible, "What Claire?"

Frumpy also never acknowledged the fact that I was the only one on her team to maintain a 0 percent redo rate, even though it was documented so everyone knew. No one else even came close to 0 percent. That's why 10 percent was set as a goal. But, of course, Frumpy could never admit that the pretty blonde was efficient.

After work, my evening hours were spent playing board games and reading to Greyson. Of course, by the time he was in kindergarten, he was able to read perfectly, but he still enjoyed being read to. After I tucked Greyson in, Sam and I often spoke on the phone. We also went on a couple more dates. I really did enjoy talking to him. He was pretty smart for a baby gorilla. In fact, he was like a walking encyclopedia. For all you young'uns out there, an encyclopedia is an actual physical book that us old folks used to retrieve information from. Sam would constantly state little facts about things on topic. We'd be at an Italian restaurant, and he'd say something like, "Did you know there are over 600 different varieties of pasta?" I couldn't decide if that was endearing or annoying or weird.

On our third date, I didn't think I could keep milking him for nice dinners without giving something in return, so I figured, *I guess I can muster up a kiss.*

It was the end of the night and we were chatting in the parking lot of my apartment. My heart was pounding as I stood there leaning against my car, waiting for an unsatisfactory kiss. *Wait. What if I've forgotten how to kiss? Or what if we lean the same way? Ugh. Please just let it be over quickly.*

As predicted, he went in for the kiss.

Mmm . . . I stand corrected.

Sam was a good kisser—not Michael Hutchence good, mind you, but pretty damn good. I'd give him a solid B+, maybe even an A-. But then I did something weird. Not him, me. . . . I laughed. I just started giggling for no apparent reason. I tried so hard to stop. *Why am I laughing? Is it because I'm kissing someone I'm not attracted to? Is it a nervous laugh? Has it just been too long since I've kissed anyone? Stop laughing!* Sam looked at me as if to say, "Did I do something funny?" and I looked at him like, "It's not you, it's me."

I apologized profusely and said it had just been so long since I'd kissed someone, and I really wasn't sure why I'd laughed. That was probably the truth. Probably.

Even though I laughed at Sam (and knew that couldn't be a good sign), we continued to date. He was so chivalrous. He always opened the door for me, pulled out my chair, let me order first, gave me his coat, and insisted on picking up the check. He even made sure he always walked on the street side of the sidewalk as if his little body could protect me from a runaway car. I hadn't been treated this gallantly since Dante. And when Sam did all these things for me, I believed it was out of sincerity, not because he wanted to get in my pants.

After a few months of dating Sam, I actually started having feelings for him. His gorillaness didn't seem to bother me anymore. The little facts and figures he told me became interesting. And his height was perfect for kissing. I didn't even laugh anymore.

Sam was also great with Greyson. During Sam's tiny window of time with Greyson, which was only when he'd pick me up for dates or drop me off, he'd do cheesy but cute magic tricks that usually ended with Greyson keeping a quarter. Greyson ate it up. I'm sure he would've smiled, if he knew how.

I waited months to let Sam actually spend time with Greyson. I told Sam that around Greyson, he was only a friend. I always knew I would never lead Greyson on with a man in his life unless it became extremely serious. Even with Sam's extremely limited exposure to Greyson and me never mentioning his diagnoses, he still figured out that Greyson was not a typical child.

Well, it didn't take a genius to figure it out. When Sam picked me up for our dates, I'd say goodbye to Greyson by holding his hands and kneeling down in front of him so we were at eye level. "Greyson, Mommy is going to dinner with a friend. Sarah is here to watch over you and do Legos with you while I'm gone. When I leave, I want you to be brave like Batman and be extra good for Sarah while Mommy is gone."

As I spoke, Greyson's eyes would look as far off to the side as physically possible while I looked directly at him.

"K."

"Okay, Greyson, so when I walk out this door, you are going to have lots of fun with Sarah, and Mommy will come home later and kiss you goodnight."

"K."

"I love you so much."

"Love you too, Mommy."

Greyson typically did better when I "precorrected" his behavior, meaning that I corrected any bad behavior before he even attempted it. This was a skill that I'd always used, but Natalie from Minnesota helped me perfect it.

After dating Sam for four months, I finally let him spend a day with both Greyson and me. We went to a festival with rides and live shows. *Please let Greyson behave. Please let Greyson behave.*

The first half of the day went okay. Generally, Greyson's behavior was better with interesting stimuli around to keep his brain active, which was one way that he didn't fit the typical autism mold. But when Sam bought Greyson tickets for the rides, I knew that spelled trouble. Greyson was deathly afraid of rides, but he agreed to try the motorcycles. You know, the little ones that just go around slowly in a circle. They don't go up and down; they don't go back and forth; they're completely stationary outside of going around a circle at about one mile an hour. There were babies on the ride, so I felt hopeful.

Greyson got on the blue motorcycle—his favorite color— and I said a little prayer. *Please Lord help Greyson make it through this ride. Please Lord, pleeeeeeease.*

When the ride began at the speed of a sloth, Greyson wrapped his arms tightly around the top of the motorcycle instead of holding the handlebars. There was a look of horror on his reddened face like he knew if he let go, he would plunge twelve inches to his death. The babies and toddlers on the ride were giggling, honking their horns, and waving gleefully to their parents. Greyson was the only kid over age two on the ride. He was also very tall for his age, so he looked like he was about seven.

Greyson then started crying hysterically. *Oh no.* And screaming. *Oh Lord.* At the top of his lungs. *Oh shit.* The teenager running the ride didn't know what to do. Clearly Greyson was not in any danger. People were staring at me like, "What the hell is wrong with your child?" I was used to this look by now, but I wasn't used to this look while with a man. I got a knot in my stomach and wanted to cry.

Greyson almost fell off the ride as it came to the opposite of a screeching halt. He ran to me as he continued crying hysterically like he'd been kidnapped and tortured for years and we were finally being reunited. I took him to a bench and tried to calm him down, but it was no use. Time was the only thing that could calm him down. I asked Sam for some water, not because I was thirsty, not because Greyson would drink in that state, but because I couldn't handle the inevitable hypothesis Sam was formulating about my parenting. *Certainly a good mother would never rear a child who behaved like this,* he must've been thinking. *Clearly she never followed through with any disciplinary structure. Obviously, Greyson was the product of horrible parenting. Doesn't she know the first thing about raising a child?*

Sam returned twenty minutes later with some water. I knew it would take a while with the crazy long lines, and that's exactly what I was counting on. But Greyson was still in hysterics.

"Can I do anything to help?" Sam asked so sweetly. He wasn't even acting embarrassed by Greyson's erratic behavior.

"No, he just needs time to calm down."

"Okay."

I'm sure Sam picked up on all the looks of judgment from the passersby as I held Greyson. He had become too big for me to carry to a secluded location. Plus, the festival was so large and so crowded that I didn't even know where we could go. I certainly wasn't taking Greyson into a port-a-potty. Ew.

Greyson finally got settled, then, in typical Greyson fashion, acted like nothing had ever happened. "Can we go play a game, Mommy?" he asked.

"I'm *game* if you are!" Sam said cheerfully. Did I mention he had cheesy jokes too?

"Sure," I said quietly with my eyes looking downward.

I thought Sam would've been long gone after witnessing what his possible future son was like. But it was quite the contrary. In fact, over our next couple dates he reminded me how much he loved me and told me he thought I was a remarkable mom. The only other man who had said that to me was my dad. Of course, no other man had seen my parenting firsthand. My dad thought his own mother, who we lovingly referred to as Pinky, walked on water. Which she did. She was a remarkable woman. I'll never forget the day my dad told me he thought I was an even better mom than Pinky. To this day, that's the highest compliment I've ever received.

A couple weeks later, Sam showed up at my apartment holding a piece of paper. I took it from him and examined it. He'd had a complete blood test and on the paper were the results. He was proving that he didn't have any sexually transmitted diseases. I told him that I wouldn't touch him without that paperwork, so apparently, Sam was ready to be touched. To be fair, the next week I had a complete blood test and showed him my paperwork too.

So there we were, a couple of HIV-negative, herpes-free

adults who had been dating for over four months. How 'bout that?

Oh no. What if I laugh after sex? What if I laugh during sex? What if he's really bad in bed? What if I'm really bad in bed? That's not possible, I've become way too much of an overachiever. What if I don't have an orgasm? What if he doesn't have an orgasm? That's not possible, I bet he'll last three minutes.

Sam was seriously the least sexy man I'd ever dated, so I figured there was no way he could be any good. A man who told corny jokes, reported obscure facts, and did cheesy magic tricks, by law, could not be good in bed.

The next time Sam and I went on a date, we went to dinner then to his house. I had never been to his house before since Sam always picked me up and dropped me off at my apartment. When we got there, his house was very . . . clean. Decorated like a dude, but immaculate. He had an old home in a very upscale Chicago suburb, so the house had a lot of character—I mean, like an all-brick exterior, original hardwood floors, and crown molding. It was a charming little house. He told me that he'd redone all the electrical and plumbing in the house since it was old.

"You did all that yourself?"

"Yeah, and I refinished these floors, knocked out a wall that was here, and fixed all the foundational cracks. Oh, and I finished the basement. I like tinkering."

"Pretty impressive." *You have no idea how horny you just made me.*

We made our way into the bedroom because that's all the foreplay I needed.

This isn't *Fifty Shades of Grey,* so I'll cut to the chase. We did not have sex-sex that night, but we did do everything else, and I learned a couple things. Number one: Shoe size is NOT a determining factor of penis size. (Come to think of it, Dante had small feet too.) Sam might have been hairy like a gorilla, but he was hung like a horse. I'm adding Dutch to my dickdar under the enormous section. Seeing Sam naked almost made me laugh—but in a good way this time—because it was so comical seeing a little man with a foot-long penis. Number two: Sam was an oral sex god. He took me to a place I didn't know existed. I had so many orgasms it brought me to tears. That time instead of laughing, I cried.

"Are you okay? Are you . . . crying?"

Covering my face with my hands and struggling to speak, I slowly mumble between my fingers, "I'm, uh (long pause), I'm (longer pause), I don't know (insanely long pause as I try to bring myself back to earth) . . . recovering."

A week later and a month shy of my six-month rule, I just couldn't resist anymore. I went to Sam's house with the intention of having sex for the first time in almost seven years. I was hoping I'd be pleasantly surprised like I was in the oral sex department (understatement of the universe).

I attacked Sam like . . . well . . . like I hadn't had sex in almost seven years. We ripped off each other's clothes while making out and staggering our way to the bedroom. He threw me on top of him and handled my body like he was a man with a short fuse and I was a vending machine that just stole his last dollar—tossing me, turning me, grabbing me, bouncing me, shaking me, slamming me up and down on his mammoth-sized penis. That was not the soft, sweet, caressing sex I had envisioned from Sam. It was way, way, WAY better. I had orgasm after orgasm after orgasm after orgasm. I kept screaming and shaking because my body wouldn't let me keep it inside. It was like every nerve ending in my body went to my vagina, and I felt like I had no bones, no weight, and no inhibitions. Sam effortlessly took complete control of my body like a ragdoll. After my—oh, I don't know—tenth orgasm, I started crying uncontrollably. Eventually my body just curled up and collapsed on top of him. And I just cried and cried. I had never cried during sex before.

Sam and I had knockdown, drag-out, insanely orgasmic, uninhibited, shamelessly violent, wild-animals-attacking-their-prey sex every weekend for a month.

And then this happened.

MICHAEL, PART TWO

2000

I was over six months into my job, into Sam, and into Chicago. Life was good—great actually—the best it'd been since my years with Anna. I was no longer depressed. And I'd acquired a sense of humor that I never knew I had. I became fucking *hilarious*. Maybe the ignite button was deep in my pussy where no one had ever gone. I finally felt happy.

I was at work and on my way to get coffee at the other end of the building with Heather, a coworker I'd befriended from the sales department. We were walking and laughing, likely making fun of Frumpy because Heather didn't like her either. As we walked through the corridor, we noticed a new desk strangely placed in the middle of nothingness, as if someone had said, "Sit here for a moment while I figure out where the hell I'm going to put you." There was a man sitting at the desk with his back facing the walkway. I didn't recognize him, but being the cheerful, friendly, newly hilarious woman I was, I decided to say hello to the new mystery man in the marketing department.

"Hi!" I said gleefully.

The mystery man slowly spun his chair around while looking down, as if he were trying to decide whether he wanted his emergence to be shy or grand. As he slowly looked up, my heart dropped into my stomach. I'm pretty sure my mouth hung open. His eyes were light green, his lips were smooth and full, his hair was dark and slicked back. He looked like he'd stepped out of *GQ* with his silver tie, pressed shirt, and polished shoes. He had a slight, sexy stubble on his face. He smelled delicious like I could lick him and eat him up. His dress shirt hugged his muscular body in all the right places.

"Hi," he said much more sexily, but far less cheerfully, than me.

"Hi." *Crap, I already said that.*

He just smiled. Holy fuck his smile was perfect. His teeth were straight and glistening white. I think I saw them twinkle like in cartoons.

(Awkward silence while I gawked.)

Heather nudged me.

"Are you new?" I spewed. *Duh. Like I wouldn't have noticed you before.*

"Yes, it's my first day. They're trying to find a spot for me." He nudged his head toward his new female boss whom I'd never met.

Um, didn't Boss Lady know Gorgeous Man was starting today? Who's this guy's new boss, and how the hell did she not know he was starting today? I assumed Boss Lady was too busy washing, waxing, shaving, brushing, primping, curling, and perfuming herself to realize, *Oh, wait a second . . . maybe Gorgeous Man will need a place to . . . I don't know . . . sit!*

"Looks like she's prepared," I joked because that's how I roll now.

"Appears that way. (Sexy pause while looking right into

my eyes.) I'm Michael by the way," he said as he extended his hand for me to shake.

Please let me be hearing things, his name cannot *be Michael.*

"Claire. Nice to meet you."

He turned to Heather and extended his hand, "Michael."

Yep. Clear as day.

"I'm Heather. Nice to meet you."

"Nice to meet you both."

"Whatcha workin' on?" I asked because I thought it was strange he had pictures of food on his screen.

"I'm working on a piece for the company's cafeteria."

"That explains it."

"Explains what?"

"The food on your screen. I'm a foodie, so I thought you were . . . I don't know, looking up food stuff or something." *Stupid, stupid, stupid Claire.*

He let out a pity laugh, "No, they put me to work already. I'm a senior graphic designer."

"Oh."

Heather chimed in, "Well, it was great meeting you. I'm sure we'll see you around."

We exchanged goodbyes, and Heather and I continued down the corridor. We weren't even three steps away before Heather exhaled and said, "Fuck, he's hot!"

"Yeah." *Fuck.*

A few weeks went by and my amazing sex-filled, orgasm-filled life continued. I stayed away from Gorgeous Man as much as humanly possible. When we'd pass in the walkway, I'd smile and say, "Hi!" then think to myself, *Don't even think about it! Don't even think about it! Don't even think about it!*

Then, one day, Gorgeous Man walked down the aisle where my cubicle was. As he walked past my desk, I couldn't help but notice he had the most beautiful ass I had ever seen in my life.

COME ON, Lord. Please stop tormenting me!

He stopped to talk to someone a few cubicles in front of mine, giving me an extended view of his yummy ass. Before he walked off, he glanced back at me and gave me a slight, sexy smile.

Don't even think about it! Don't even think about it! Don't even think about it. You love Sam. You love Sam.

Not long after, everyone in the marketing department received an e-mail stating that the graphic artists had been reassigned to accommodate our growing number of catalogs. I was in charge of all Venture catalogs, and up until then, Kimberly was the graphic artist assigned to my catalogs. All was good. We were comfortable and worked perfectly fine together, so I wasn't happy to hear they were restructuring. As I scrolled down the e-mail, I saw that all Venture catalogs were reassigned to . . . I'll give you one guess. Yep. Gorgeous Man.

No, no, no, no, no! Anyone but him. Lord, now you're just being cruel.

This news meant that I'd be working intimately with Gorgeous Man.

This can't be good. And I should probably start calling him Michael. Jesus take the wheel!

Michael and I had a late morning meeting to discuss how we'd move forward as a team in the production process of our Venture catalogs. I didn't remember a single word from our meeting because he was too damn dreamy. We decided to continue our meeting over lunch. But of course, over lunch we talked about life more than work. I told him about Sam.

There. I did it. I am off-limits. No touchy.

Michael told me all about his baby nephew in a sickeningly adorable way. *Let me guess, you have a little puppy and volunteer at a soup kitchen in your free time. Stop the madness!*

Luckily, no puppy or volunteer work came up, but he sure was crazy about his little nephew. There's got to be something about you that's not perfect. Well, his name *was* Michael, just like Sperm Donor. (Insert vomit emoji.) And I did vow never to date another Michael. Unfortunately, that rule wasn't holding enough water. *Why are there so many fucking Michaels in the world?*

A month into working with Michael, everything was going great—a little too great. We flirted with one another relentlessly and made each other laugh like crazy. He was so goofy. He didn't look like the goofy type, but he definitely had the goof factor. I started thinking about Michael—and not just because we had another meeting scheduled or because we had to review our catalog before submission, but because I couldn't make myself stop thinking about him. And boy, did I try. I tried so hard to keep Michael out of my head. *Sam,* I would remind myself, *you're in love with Sam. Thinks-you-walk-on-water-best-sex-in-the-universe Sam.*

Sam and I were still going strong and our incredible sex was unwavering. There aren't words in the English language to describe how incredible our sex was. But then I started to think to myself, *Maybe* I'm *the one who's amazing in bed. Maybe* I'm *the reason why my body collapses and I break into tears when we're done. Maybe I'm just* that *good. I mean, maybe I just don't realize how unbelievably talented I am. I was so young and inexperienced when I got pregnant, so I never discovered my inner sexual goddess. Sam sure is lucky to have met me after my full transformation from ordinary being to extraordinarily sexual being. Sam . . . you're welcome.*

. . .

My employer scheduled semiannual "team-building" events for the marketing department. *Gag.* Frumpy only attended these events out of her managerial duties because I'm pretty sure she couldn't care less about building her team's camaraderie. She'd never even looked at me, except the three times I sat in her chair for thirty minutes begging for acknowledgment. *Hey, Frumps, it's me, Claire, the invisible girl with the 0 percent redo rate for the past eight months.*

The first marketing event after Michael came on board was held at a sports bar. I begrudgingly headed there because my favorite people in the company weren't in the marketing department and the last thing my relationship with Sam needed was away-from-work time with Michael. He was the only person in marketing who was any fun.

So I went to the sports bar, and Michael and I just sat there making fun of Frumpy and her dowdy ways. There were a few other easy targets in marketing that we made fun of to help us pass the time at our "team-building" event. Since alcohol was involved, we sat there cracking up at our hilarity at the expense of others. It was pretty fun, actually. Michael always made me laugh out loud. Sam never made me laugh out loud. When Michael went to grab us another round of drinks, I watched him from across the room. While he waited for our drinks, he chatted with some other guys in the department. I just sat there, watching him. At one point, Michael laughed at something one of the other guys said. He had the best smile. I just sat there watching him smile. Then he did this thing when he laughed, where he shyly covered his mouth with his hand while slightly lifting his shoulders like he had a secret. He did that sometimes. And I just sat there, watching him with his little secret, thinking to myself, *The woman who marries that man will be the luckiest woman in the world.*

A RESORT, A CHAUFFEUR, AND
FIFTY DOLLAR DOG SHAMPOO

2000–2001

*G*reyson finished kindergarten, but not on a good note. Phone calls were made, conferences were held, and meetings took place. They told me Greyson would have to go to an alternative school for first grade because he was unable to function appropriately within a general education classroom. (Painful sigh.) My kindergartner was kicked out of school—again.

Not knowing what to do—or maybe just ignoring the fact that I had a son with autism, sensory processing disorder, and oppositional defiant disorder—I decided to move out of the school district. Perhaps they just didn't understand my son. Perhaps Greyson just had two crappy kindergarten teachers. Perhaps all the professionals who sat in all those meetings discussing him were just overrated government employees who didn't give a shit. Why couldn't they see that he was extraordinary? They gave Greyson a zillion tests and he scored in the ninety-ninth percentile in all academic areas. Didn't they know Albert Einstein was rebellious toward authority, had extreme tantrums, and was kicked out of multiple schools? Did they really want to be known as the school that kicked out the next Albert Einstein?

I found a new shitty apartment right next to my work. Unfortunately, my job was located in an affluent area, so I got a much worse apartment for much higher rent. I also had to pay an outrageous fee for breaking my lease. I thought it would be worth it to eliminate my long commute, gain two extra hours with Greyson each day, and dodge the alternative school bullet. I missed having so much time with Greyson like I did the first five years of his life. During his kindergarten year, I'd worked for Queen Linda, then I gained a two-hour commute and a social life, so my time with Greyson lessened. Maybe that's why he was being so naughty. Two more hours with Greyson every day would help, I just knew it.

I moved into my new shithole. It felt like my entire life was shifting again—like God didn't know what to do with me. I was transitioning between apartments and transitioning between men. I was still dating Sam, but my feelings for Michael kept growing. No matter how wonderful Sam was, no matter how fantastic our sex life was, no matter how accepting Sam was of Greyson, I just couldn't get Michael out of my head. Even though I never acted on my feelings for Michael, Sam was beginning to notice that something was off. My feelings and actions toward Sam started diminishing, and he sensed I was distancing myself from him. So he did what any madly-in-love man would do: he proposed.

But he not only proposed, he proposed with the most beautiful ring I'd ever seen. It was an antique style (my favorite) with so many gorgeous, intricate details surrounding a big rock. It had to be at least a two-carat diamond solitaire in the center. It was gorgeous. But he had to know that he was proposing to a woman he was losing. I didn't know what to say, so I told him I'd think about it—just what every man wants to hear after a proposal.

I called Michael crying because that's what every woman does after being proposed to by another man. I felt so confused, and ironically, I felt like Michael was my closest friend. I told him Sam proposed, and then I confessed that I think about him a lot—like a lot, a lot. He told me he thought about me too and that he loved me. I felt like God was playing a trick on me, like He was saying, "Ha ha, hee-hee! I had men ignore you for six years, and now I have them fighting over you. Isn't that hysterical?"

I took a few days off work to clear my head and examine my life. Sam was the answer to all my problems. He was kind. He was successful. He would make a great dad. He could rebuild a freaking house. He had a foot-long penis. What else could a woman ask for?

Just.

Say.

Yes.

Say yes, say yes, say YES. What the hell is wrong with you?

JUST SAY YES.

I tried to say yes. I wanted to say yes. I practiced saying yes. But I kept thinking to myself, *I can't say yes when I'm thinking about another man.* I imagined myself walking down the aisle pretending Sam was Michael. That couldn't be right. I should've been excited, not contemplating my answer. Sam deserved to marry someone who was excited to marry him, not someone who was thinking about someone else. I couldn't say yes.

There were tears, there was confusion, and I knew I was making the wrong decision as the words left my mouth, but I told Sam no. And that was that. I got a taste of a fairy-tale ending and willingly threw it all in the garbage to date Rico

Suave. I was beginning to think I was incapable of making a good decision.

First grade in a new district began for Greyson. So calls were rolling in, behavioral tests were being administered, and meetings were being scheduled. I ignorantly thought I could beat the system by moving Greyson to another district. As if his old schools would never mail their inch-thick file on Greyson to the new school. Like Greyson would magically conform to his new school's expectations and his teacher would see him as a challenging yet miraculous gift in her life like I did.

I went to my first big meeting at Greyson's new school, and it was the same old information, just in a different location.

"Greyson is brilliant. Greyson scored at the ninety-ninth percentile here, here, here, here, and here. But Greyson cannot control his outbursts, so students have repeatedly evacuated the classroom. Greyson's behavior in the classroom is extremely defiant."

Greyson bad. Other kids good. Grrr.

As I sat in that starchy white room with fluorescent lights and cheap vinyl flooring, I could feel the judgment. I've voiced my opinion that the most judgmental people in the world are born-again Christians, but teachers hold the silver medal when it comes to judging parents. I felt like standing up in that heartless room and screaming, "First of all, I had a perfect diet when I was pregnant because I loved Greyson before he was born. Next, I saw five lactation specialists and ultimately nursed Greyson for over a year because bonding and all the health benefits were *that* important to me. I never put Greyson down when he was a baby—I cuddled him, rocked him, sang to him, and smothered him with kisses every day. I made Greyson homemade baby food because I knew exactly what was in it. I didn't work during the first two years of his life, but I did earn a degree—just like you bozos—in early childhood education, and, by the way, I only studied when Greyson was asleep because I wanted as much time with him as possible. I've told Greyson I love him every day of his life. I don't physically, psychologically, or verbally abuse him, even though you're looking at me like I do. I've read the books and done *EVERYTHING* they said to do. I put handwritten notes (with stickers dammit!) in Greyson's perfectly packed, healthy lunch every day. I've prayed to God every day. I've asked Him to protect Greyson and thanked Him for blessing me with a complex, brilliant, and unique child. Furthermore, I love Greyson unconditionally. No mother has ever loved a child more than I love Greyson. No mother has ever tried harder to be a great mom than me. So stop talking to me like an uneducated, meth-making mom, and stop looking at me with your pitiful looks. In conclusion, fuck you, you, you, you, you, you, you, and you."

Well, that was what I *wanted* to say, but instead I sat there and nodded like they were insightful and brilliant. The meeting concluded and the decision was made to "temporarily" send Greyson to an alternative school.

And then there were three.

My six-year-old son was kicked out of three schools, I just dumped the man I thought I would marry, and I lived in a shithole apartment. Perfect.

Naturally, Michael and I became an instant item after I waived my right to a white picket fence with Sam. Plus, Michael had already professed his love to me. As soon as we began our relationship, I questioned what would become of us. Men that good-looking can't stay faithful. They can't make a commitment like marriage. God put them on this planet to look at, not to marry. Sam had the words *marriage material* written all over him while Michael had the words *commitment phobic playa* written all over him—even though he had never said or done anything around me to make me feel that way. It was just common sense really. Nice guys don't come in smoking-hot packages.

Word must've gotten to Frumpy that Michael and I were an item, and she didn't approve of us dating. I always thought Frumpy had the hots for Michael—but I mean, who wouldn't —but it was weird because she looked like she couldn't even spell the word *sex*. And surprisingly, she was actually married to a man, who I assumed must be blind and deaf. Once Frumpy got word of my relationship with Michael, she started being even ruder to me. She used to just make me wait for thirty minutes to ask a question, never acknowledged my 0 percent redo rate, and ignored my never-missed-a-single-deadline performance. After she found out about Michael and me, she added other things to her repertoire, like rolling her eyes at me, making backhanded comments about me, and looking at the floor when I walked by.

Despite the turmoil at work, things were going well with Michael. We had the same sense of humor, so we cracked each other up. Basically, we were the same amount of crazy. I still missed Sam, but not nearly as much as I'd anticipated, so yay for that. I think I just missed sex since I had to start over with my stupid sixish-month rule. *Why can't I have a third-date rule like everyone else?* Although, nowadays there seems to be a no-date rule, which is so gross to me. All I see on TV now is people having sex twelve minutes after they meet, and it terrifies me as a mother that this is the new norm. Once in a while, I'd like to see a follow-up show on how those one-night stands led to herpes, hepatitis, HIV, or all three.

It was the year 2000, and an HIV test wasn't considered 100 percent accurate until six months after exposure. Every time I spoke with Anna on the phone, it reminded me to be careful, especially since I was a mom. Anna was perpetually on my mind, but sadly, we didn't talk much anymore. She usually refused my calls or her parents refused them for her. "Anna nie może mówić (Anna can't talk)," was all they would say. And I couldn't just show up at their house because I had no idea where they lived. They understandably wanted privacy during that heartbreaking time. When they did hand the phone to Anna, she sounded miserably weak and delusional. After our conversations, I'd curl up on the floor and cry. To this day, Anna was the greatest friend I've ever had.

Christmastime was approaching, and Greyson was acclimated to his new alternative school. The good news was that the phone calls and meetings stopped because all the kids were naughty at this school. I was heading to his school for the first time for a holiday performance. I had never been there before because the school was really far away, and strangely, Greyson was picked up and dropped off by a taxicab each day. Greyson was the only student the driver picked up, so basically he had his own personal driver. When she arrived the first day, I was like, "Do I pay you?" and she was like, "No ma'am." Okay. Superweird. Of course I gave her a generous Christmas gift like I always did with Greyson's teachers and now his, um, chauffeur.

I arrived at his school early and slowly walked down the hallway toward the gym where the performance would take place. As I snooped, I mean walked painstakingly slowly down the hallway, I looked through all the windows and open doors to the classrooms. A feeling of panic and helplessness overtook me as I watched students moaning, screaming, rocking, spinning, crying, and being restrained.

There must be different rules regarding restraining students at this type of school, I thought. *Maybe it's because the teachers have a special education certificate and additional training, but I'm not sure.* As I continued to walk, I didn't see any schoolwork in progress. I felt a pit in my stomach thinking Greyson had been severely misplaced—like in the movies when someone accidentally gets trapped in a mental institution and can't get out.

The school had an Olympic-sized indoor swimming pool and a recreation room to work on their gross motor skills. Of course, Greyson loved that he got to swim and play in the recreation room every day. Between the swimming pool and the chauffeur, I think Greyson believed his school was a resort. But because Greyson was unable to pick up on social cues, he didn't realize that he was surrounded by children with mental illness.

After the performance, I met his teacher. I summoned my fake smile and said, "Great job with the performance!" *Total lie, it wasn't that great.*

"Thank you! And Greyson is doing a wonderful job in school." That was a first. "Boy, is he smart!"

Yeah, I know. "Thanks. Um, speaking of Greyson, do you, um, think this school is a good fit for him?"

"Absolutely! He fits right in."

Not the answer I was looking for. "Soooo, you think Greyson's behavior is suited for a school setting like this?"

A little less cheery this time because I think she knew what I was digging for. "Yes, Greyson has been appropriately placed in our program."

"Oh." The smile drained from my face.

"I know it's a little hard to take in at first, but I assure you, Greyson is where he should be."

"Oh." I mumbled trying to hold back my tears. "Okay. Thank you."

When I got back in my car, I cried the whole way home. Greyson couldn't belong there. He just couldn't.

The holidays had come and gone, and I was back at work. Frumpy was so sweet to take a moment to thank me for the generous gift basket I got her from a very popular, expensive, Chicago-based bath and body store.

"The shower gel smells so good. We washed our dog with it."

(Insert eyes bulging out of head emoji.) "You washed . . . your dog . . . with my gift?" *Do you have any idea what I paid for that?!*

"Yeah, well actually, my husband didn't know what it was, so he washed the dog with it, and now she smells really good."

"Oh, okay. Glad your dog is enjoying your gift." *What a bitch . . . you, not the dog.*

That may be the rudest thing anyone has ever said to me. Didn't Frumpy realize that I was a single mom trying to survive on a crappy paycheck with no help and no child support? And I never bought things like that for myself because I couldn't afford it? I bought it for her because she's my boss—if you can call a person who has never helped, guided, or encouraged me in any way, shape, or form a boss. And that's what a good employee does—gives a nice Christmas present to her shitty boss.

Michael cheered me up with a nice evening out—steak dinner and a movie. *Mmm . . . steak.* He knew food was the way to my heart. We sat on the same side of the booth like all annoyingly adorable couples do. We snuggled and chatted the night away.

My mom and dad, who were still in town from the holidays, were watching Greyson, so I spent the night at Michael's place. I never once let Sam or Michael spend the night at my place because I didn't want to set a bad example for Greyson.

Michael and I were approaching the sixth-month mark, and he'd already furnished his prerequisite pre-sex documentation. He was herpes-, hepatitis-, and HIV-free. To my young readers, neither Sam nor Michael hesitated for a moment when I asked for this paperwork. If you ever date someone who calls this request ridiculous—run! They're not worth it and may infect you with a deadly disease. A stand-up guy, or gal, will happily get a blood test for you. Take care of your body because no one is worth jeopardizing your health and your life. Take it from Anna.

After dinner, Michael and I headed back to his place to watch the movie *Where the Heart Is*. It was our first movie together because we could never agree on one. He's more a *Shawshank Redemption, Gladiator, Braveheart* kinda guy, and I'm more a *When Harry Met Sally, Pretty Woman, Miss Congeniality* kinda gal. Although we later found out we're both *Tommy Boy, Liar Liar,* and *Happy Gilmore* kinda folks. Unlike Sam, Michael was not the type to suffer through a chick flick for my benefit. I did miss Sam's willingness to do anything for me.

The movie was amazing, even though I found out that Michael only watched it to look at Natalie Portman. That's okay because I couldn't keep my eyes off her either. When the movie was over I said, "I love the name Novalee. I've never heard it before." (That was Natalie Portman's character's name in the movie.) Michael responded, "That is a nice name. I like it too." So we could agree on names. Good to know.

We worked our way into the bedroom buzzed on wine

and Natalie Portman. We ripped off each other's clothes and proceeded to do the deed. FINALLY.

The sex was . . . good. Like normal people sex good. I had an orgasm, but not twelve. Maybe it was first-time sex jitters. Or maybe, just maybe, I'm actually *not* a sex goddess.

Nah.

GOODBYE, HELLO, GOODBYE

2001

*B*y January 2001, I'd been at my job a year and was still maintaining a flawless record without a speck of acknowledgment from my boss. And then, it finally happened: an all-marketing e-mail went out stating that I was "Employee of the Quarter." Typically, when those e-mails went out, the person's boss wrote a long paragraph about all the wonderful qualities said employee held and all their amazing accomplishments. But no, not for me. I got one sentence.

"Congratulations to our Employee of the Quarter, Claire, who has maintained a 0 percent redo rate for a year."

Wow Frumps, that was so fucking heartwarming. You forgot to mention the "never missed a deadline" part, the "works well with others" part, the "has a positive attitude" part, and the "always willing to go the extra mile" part. It must've eaten her up inside sending that out. My guess was that Frump's boss made her do it. Bite me, Frumps.

. . .

A few weeks later, in February 2001, I was sitting at my desk when the phone rang. "Hello, this is Claire, how may I help you?" I said with a smile because I read you can hear whether a person is smiling over the phone.

"Hi Claire. It's Anna's brother."

Oh no. "Hi," I whispered, my smile deflating.

"Anna passed. I know she'd like you at her service."

"I'm so sorry. Of course. Of course, I'll be at her service."

"It's this Friday at nine thirty at Kopec Reszke Funeral Home in Chicago."

"Okay. I'll be there. Thanks for letting me know."

"Bye."

"Bye."

I ran out of the building, trudged across the icy parking lot, and slumped into my frozen car. I shivered and cried hysterically while mascara bled down my face and my nose dripped onto my dress. For hours, I just listened to the wind push against my windows and the heater chug.

I couldn't believe Anna was gone. I'd never even said goodbye. The world had no idea what it had just lost. She would've done so much good. She would've been a star—a star who used her influence to help others rather than herself. But instead, she was gone forever. I'd never find another friend like Anna, and life would never be the same. I had a giant hole in my heart and thought about Anna every single day. Sometimes every hour, sometimes every minute. Between Anna passing and Sperm Donor leaving me to raise Greyson by myself, I didn't know how much more I could handle.

Shortly after Anna passed, I decided to reach out to Sperm Donor's sister, Mary, who lived in Oklahoma. I got Mary's phone number from Sperm Donor's stepmom, who I decided to check in with for no good reason other than I'm a glutton for punishment. Perhaps I was in search of someone to fill an open position in Greyson's life. He didn't have a father and now he didn't have a godmother. I'd never met Mary, and I knew nothing about her except that her brother was the devil.

Mary and I had a very awkward conversation that ended in her saying, "I'll be in Chicago on business next week. Can we get together?" *Whoa, hold your horses, Spanky. I wasn't expecting to go from zero to sixty at hello. Perhaps I should've thought this through.*

Well, it wasn't Mary's fault that her brother had the integrity of a rat. Perhaps meeting Mary would be good for Greyson, although Greyson had never once asked about his father. Maybe he never picked up on the social norm that it was conventional to have a mom *and* a dad. Greyson never asked, but about twice a year I'd say, "Greyson, you know, if you ever have any questions about your father, you can talk to me." He always responded with an indifferent, "Okay."

A huge pet peeve of mine is when divorced parents talk smack about one another to their kids. I'll never understand why parents burden their children with their emotional drama and hold their hate for one another in higher regard than their love for their children. Sperm Donor and I were never married, but the same rule applied. I'd never once mentioned to Greyson what a pathetic loser Sperm Donor was. Plus, it'd be much more fun to write a book. Luckily, not speaking poorly about Sperm Donor was easier than anticipated because Greyson literally never once asked about him. I wrote Greyson a letter when he was a baby telling him all the things I loved about Sperm Donor. I wanted Greyson to know he was conceived out of love and that I'd loved his dad very much.

So after not nearly enough deliberation, I thought, *What the hell . . . I'll meet up with Mary.*

Big, big, big mistake.

I still get a sick feeling when I think about our day together. What should have been a nice day of getting to know each other ended up being a day full of overwhelming emotions. All the sadness, confusion, panic, heartbreak, rejection, and fear I experienced when Sperm Donor left me came crashing back. I didn't know how to act, what to say, what to do.

The three of us went out to lunch. As I sat across from Mary, I did my best to avoid eye contact. I frantically filled every lull in our conversation with asinine comments, like it was my first time talking to another human. That day, my social awkwardness made a bigger comeback than Neil Patrick Harris after *Doogie Howser*.

During lunch, Greyson just quietly read a book. He was completely oblivious that Mary was his aunt. Somewhere in between my moronic remarks, I did learn one interesting fact: Mary told me Sperm Donor had impregnated and left yet another woman. Now Greyson had a half sister *and* a half brother—that we knew of.

After lunch, we went to the Lego Store—where Greyson could build a village and live for eternity. I knew Greyson could hyperfocus there for hours if need be. I didn't know what to do with myself while we were there. Do I play Legos with Greyson to show Mary what a good mom I am? Do I try to recover from our disastrous lunch conversation? Whatever I did, it always felt wrong. When I played with Greyson, I felt like I was trying too hard. When I attempted a conversation with Mary, I felt like I was being too stupid. I just wanted the day to be over.

But instead, I extended it.

Later that evening, I got a sitter while Mary, her boyfriend (who'd come with her to Chicago), Michael, and I went out to dinner. Not sure where the logic was to have a double date. During dinner I made an attempt at a penis joke.

What? Who just said that? Michael thought it was hilarious because there was a compliment in it somewhere, but I was horrified. I couldn't hold my liquor, and that was a night that required liquor.

After making several failed attempts to, oh, I don't know:

Impress Mary? Ugh.

Feel accepted? Perhaps.

Get closure? Please.

Gain acknowledgment? We do exist.

Feel validated? That'd be nice.

None of the above? Affirmative.

Whatever the fuck my goal was that swirly-twirly night didn't work because Greyson and I had plans to spend the next day with Mary, and she totally stood us up. She didn't show up and never called. She left Chicago, and our lives, without a word. I guess I shouldn't have been surprised.

THE SANDWICH APPROACH

2001–2002

*M*ichael and I were going strong. We got along great. We didn't argue. We made each other laugh. He was faithful—I never worried he'd cheat on me. He was loyal—he'd had the same large, close-knit group of friends since he was four. He was a family man—he loved and took care of his parents and nephew. And finally, the sex was really, truly, very . . . good.

I came to the disappointing conclusion that I was not, in fact, a sex goddess. Hard to believe, I know—I was so certain of my goddessness. The sad realization was the only variable that distinguished the difference between good and out-of-body-experience sex was, well, Sam. I guess I didn't have enough experience to realize that sex with Sam was a gift. It was like Christian Grey, John Mayer, and women's unrealistic expectations all rolled into one. There I was, sweet, innocent, inexperienced, delusional little Claire thinking that I'd magically become a sexual mastermind after a combined total of approximately two months of sex in my life. Sex with Michael was just like sex with Sperm Donor. Good. Pleasurable. Nice. Satisfying. Fun. Singularly orgasmic. An all-around great time. A solid B+. I wish I'd never experienced sex with Sam because after a lot of girl talk with friends, I'm pretty sure sex with Sam was as likely as finding a unicorn. Both Sam and Michael were great guys, so I guess I'd traded hot sex for hot looks. I traded Sam's Claire-walks-on-water mentality for Michael's five-star baby-making genes. A year earlier, when I was making the decision between the two men, I kept thinking, *Why did God bring Michael into my life at the very moment I was about to marry Sam after being alone for so long?* I'm a strong believer that things happen for a reason. It's either that or God has a sick sense of humor.

In the fall of 2001, Greyson started second grade. I was still perturbed that no one in the universe, except my parents, seemed to understand that my genius son didn't belong at an alternative school. He belonged at an academically challenging school. I wanted him at a school where acceptable behavior was modeled by his peers, not at a school where all he saw was screaming, rocking, moaning, flailing, and outbursts. How was he supposed to transform in that environment? How was his brilliant mind being nourished? At his school, he never had homework, and I saw no evidence of schoolwork.

On a warm day in late September, as I strolled through the door to the IEP meeting I had requested based on my concern of misplacement, I was feeling desperate. An IEP is an individualized educational plan, and meetings are held to make decisions regarding special education and related services. This particular IEP meeting was held at his former school because the decision in play was whether he would be allowed to return there or not.

I took a seat in that all-too-familiar, chalky white room

with cheap fluorescent lighting, where seven people sat at an enormous rectangular table: the principal, nurse, occupational therapist, speech therapist, school psychologist, director of student services, and a teacher I didn't recognize. They were all there to represent—or should I say defend— the second grade. *Well, this isn't intimidating at all. Maybe they're all here to congratulate me on Greyson's invitation to return to their school.* (Sound the *Family Feud* X buzzer here.)

They went around and solemnly introduced themselves to me while avoiding eye contact and fidgeting with their papers like they were about to tell me I had six months to live. *Well that's not the enthusiasm I was expecting at Greyson's welcome-back party.*

"Hello. Thank you for meeting with us today to discuss Greyson's progress and placement. We're happy to report that Greyson is doing very well in the alternative program. We have communicated with the faculty at Greyson's school, and it sounds as though the alternative program has been a good fit for him."

"Okay," I said, but in my head, I was thinking: *Of course Greyson is doing well there. How hard is it to swim and play all day? Not to mention that I'm sure his behavior is pretty stellar in comparison to that of his peers, so let's cut the crap and start planning his homecoming.*

"Greyson is under constant assessment in his program, and academically, he continues to be off the charts."

"Okay." This is what teachers call the "sandwich approach:" start with a couple positive statements (bottom bun), state the actual message you want to divulge (meat and cheese), and then end on a happy note with a big fake smile (top bun). Bring on the meat and cheese in three, two, one . . .

"After careful consideration and deliberation, we, along with the teachers and specialists in Greyson's current program, have decided that Greyson would benefit from another year at the alternative school."

Bam. "So Greyson has to stay another year at the alternative school, but then he can return to this school?" *Oh, and by the way, you didn't deliberate shit.*

"At this time, we cannot state if Greyson will be ready for a traditional classroom setting in a year."

"When I went to visit the alternative school, I felt as though Greyson did not belong in the program. I don't believe he's being challenged academically and may regress socially being surrounded by students who constantly exhibit even more severe behaviors than him." *Have any of you even set foot in that school? I highly doubt it since it's a million miles away.*

"I hear your concerns, however, we cannot accommodate Greyson's needs at our school at this time. We unanimously agree that Greyson is appropriately placed in the alternative school program."

Of course you do, you don't have to deal with him there. My eyes started welling up. *Don't cry, don't cry, don't cry.*

"We know Greyson is a very sweet, special, and gifted boy, but he requires interventions that we cannot provide at our school at this time."

Top bun.

"We will reevaluate Greyson's placement in a year." Big smiles by all in attendance. Ta-da.

I left the meeting feeling powerless and confused. No one seemed to understand Greyson's astounding potential. Could you imagine Sheldon Cooper just swimming and playing for two years? Me neither.

I never admitted it to myself, but perhaps Greyson was not equipped to withstand a regular classroom. It felt like there was no place for him. There was no school for gifted kids with oppositional defiant disorder and autism. There was no place where Greyson could study chemistry in one room and beat the shit out of something in another.

Although, thankfully, Greyson's episodes had diminished significantly. In fact, he'd gone from hitting me a hundred times a day to only having severe episodes two to four times a month. He was as skinny as a string bean, so even though he always got in a few good smacks, I was still able to restrain him. Not carry him, but restrain him. He was, however, very tall. He was not as strong as the average seven-year-old because he wasn't physical. Unless you consider assembling Legos physical—he had the strongest fingers in the universe. He could assemble a 2,000-piece Lego set in a flash. And, God forbid, I helped him with his Legos. That would just slow him down, and I'd do it "all wrong."

I tried making Greyson more physical by signing him up for sports. I also thought sports would help his social skills, teach him the importance of teamwork, and help him (oh please, Lord) make just one friend. But sports didn't go so well for either of us. In baseball, he just picked grass in the outfield; in floor hockey, he just twirled his hockey stick; in soccer, he just stood there waiting for the ball to ricochet off his foot. Going to his games was excruciating, but I never let him drop out of a sport. I thought I was teaching him the importance of finishing what he started and being there for his team. Yeah, I didn't accomplish any of that. Not even the make-a-friend part. I actually think moms waited until after we'd left to hand out birthday invitations. Greyson did like snacks after the games and medals after the season. Like he deserved a medal. Please. If anyone deserved a medal it was me. I had to sit through all those practices and games in a desperate attempt to integrate my son. And trying to find a friend for Greyson or scrounge up a birthday party invitation was like nailing Jell-O to a tree. It was so aggravating because I threw a great birthday party for

Greyson every year in hopes that he'd receive an invitation in return. Since the time Greyson was in preschool, I'd invited his entire class to his parties. He'd had parties at Chuck E. Cheese, a children's museum, an arcade—one year I even rented out a small indoor water park. Moms brought their fake smiles and dropped off their children and five-dollar gifts. But no one ever invited Greyson to a birthday party in return.

My relationship with Michael continued to grow in all areas except one: the Greyson area. Michael struggled with accepting, or even liking, Greyson. He told me he was having difficulty bonding with a boy who beat me up. That broke my heart because Greyson and I were a package deal. I expected Michael to love me so much that he'd love Greyson too since he was a part of me. I refused to believe Greyson was that difficult to love. Instead of seeing Greyson's brilliance, Michael saw Greyson's defiance. Instead of seeing Greyson's potential, Michael saw Greyson's oddities. Instead of seeing my love for Greyson, Michael saw everyone's dislike for Greyson. I felt so hurt that he didn't see him the way I did. And Michael, like everyone else, didn't understand how such a good mom could raise such a bad boy.

Michael and I had been together for a year and a half and often discussed getting married. Every time the subject came up, I expressed how important it was to me that he adopt Greyson. But those conversations never ended well. In my opinion, if we got married and he didn't adopt Greyson, we wouldn't be a family. It would be different if Greyson had a father who was involved in his life (instead of the scum of the earth that he was). That was a big issue to disagree on, and it started to put a strain on our relationship.

Despite our recent tension, Michael and I were excited

about our company's annual employee event, especially since team building was not on the agenda. Every year the company rented Six Flags before it was opened to the public in the spring. It was always such a fun day because there weren't any lines since the company had the park to itself. When we arrived, Michael jumped on a few roller coasters while I watched Greyson put a death grip on the spinning ladybugs. Greyson still couldn't handle any rides that exceeded 0.001 miles per hour. I used to give him a big smile, a thumbs up, and a "Hang in there, buddy!" when he screamed bloody murder on a ride with a bunch of one-year-olds, but now that he met the height requirement for the roller coasters, it was just plain ridiculous. Greyson being extremely tall for his age made his fear look even more absurd. He looked like Buddy the Elf on toddler rides.

After enduring as much embarrassment as we could handle, we went to Greyson's favorite attraction—a giant room filled with toy guns where you shoot people with foam balls to your heart's content. Greyson could run around shooting people all day long, his face bright red and dripping with sweat. But that's totally normal for a seven-year-old, right?

At least Michael and I got to hang out and relax while Greyson gleefully obliviated any child in his path. However, having so much time to talk went terribly wrong on this fun-filled day.

"You know I love you, right?" Michael mumbled trying not to make eye contact.

"Uh, yeah," I hesitantly whispered.

"I've been thinking about you and getting married and . . . well, Greyson."

"K."

"I would marry you in a second, but I . . . I just don't see myself as Greyson's dad. I don't think I can do it. I can't adopt Greyson."

"So you've made your decision? This is your decision? You won't adopt Greyson?"

"I'm sorry. I've been thinking about this a lot, and I just can't. I don't feel a connection with Greyson the way a father should. I just can't do it. I'm sorry."

Tears filled my eyes as our conversation fell silent. I couldn't even look at him anymore. That was it, we were over, just like that. Perhaps Greyson getting put to shame by toddlers on rides and then portraying a serial killer with foam weaponry was a bit too much for one day.

So my life looked like this:

1. I had a terrible boss who ignored my achievements. By then, I had hit the two-year mark with no redos or missed deadlines. Plus, I really missed teaching.
2. I'd lost two marriage prospects—good ones.
3. I had no family in Chicago except my sister who had no involvement with Greyson or any experience with children whatsoever, yet somehow she was a parenting expert. She critiqued every move I made and every word I said during the two days I saw her per year.

But the worst part about my life at this point was that Greyson was trapped in an alternative school with absolutely no indication of returning to a traditional classroom. I contacted both schools again to see if there was any likelihood of Greyson returning to his regular school for third grade. Both schools clearly stated there was no possibility.

Now what? I loved Chicago but felt completely helpless

about Greyson's education. No matter where I lived in the Chicagoland area, Greyson would be at an alternative school. That was extremely concerning and a huge disservice to Greyson considering his academic potential. So I did what I felt was best for Greyson in that moment in his life—I moved back in with my parents in California.

Well that was a fun two years. Now back to square one.

I FINALLY DO

2002–2003

I gave two weeks' notice at work, packed up my crap, and told Michael buh-bye. While we were in Chicago, Greyson had never made a single friend or had a connection with anyone or anything. So whether we moved next door or across the country, change never seemed to bother him, which didn't align with an autism diagnosis. Greyson's episodes were triggered by little things like me telling him, "It's getting late, so let's finish the puzzle tomorrow." He was weirdly adaptable to big changes like switching schools because he got kicked out. Three times. At this point in his life, Greyson had been introduced to video games, so a cross-country drive felt like a reward. Normally, I limited his time to an hour on Saturday and Sunday only, but during this million-hour drive, I let him have at it—with the occasional, unsuccessful attempt to have him "look out the window and appreciate nature, dammit."

When we arrived in Southern California, my parents were thrilled. They were the only other humans that loved and understood Greyson the way I did. They loved him unconditionally, and together, we all turned a blind eye to his oddities. The three of us never spoke of Greyson's diagnoses. Greyson's unusual behaviors were the elephant in the room that we all turned into an adorable, pink, fluffy, lovable, flying elephant. We focused on how brilliant and handsome Greyson was and ignored the frightening facts that he never made eye contact, never smiled, never made a friend, and beat the crap out of people. *That's just Greyson, our quirky little genius!* We swept Greyson's idiosyncrasies so far under the rug that when we talked to people about him, it went something like this, "Greyson is doing wonderfully! He gets straight As in school, and he loves Legos—he can build any structure in the blink of an eye!" Since my family was scattered all over the county, no one even knew of Greyson's diagnoses. Not even Greyson. I thought if I told Greyson it would hold him back in life. I thought he'd be like, *Well, I have autism, so I'm not capable of this, this, or this.* In 2002, autism was just making its way out of the woodwork in society, and people still didn't have a clue about oppositional defiant disorder and sensory processing disorder. Plus, my parents and I believed with all our hearts that Greyson would be fine. All we had to do was love him unconditionally, shower him with happy life experiences, and nurture his brilliance, and Greyson would become hugely successful. We were sure of it.

Our ignorance was partially due to the fact that Greyson was my first child and my parents' first grandchild. We all thought Greyson's behaviors stemmed from the fact that he was a genius. You could tell he was always thinking with his cute little serious face and tense eyebrows. It was just too difficult for Greyson to relate to regular children. When kids were busy driving their Hot Wheels around making *vroom-vroom* sounds, Greyson just wanted them to shut the hell up. He wanted to figure out how Hot Wheels were made and the velocity they were capable of so he could build a meticulous track for optimum performance. And whatever you do—do not, I repeat *do not*, try to help him. Only Greyson alone could get it just right.

As much as I loved my miniature mastermind, I wished he would display just a shred of happiness. *Just one smile. A little giggle. I'd settle for a tiny grin.* Even on Christmas morning, he still didn't look happy. Although, I did manage to get a few pictures of him smiling with my mastered skill of tickle, tickle, tickle, pull arm away, grab the shot. Greyson would only smile when he was being tickled, so his face *was* physically capable of smiling.

By this time, my parents had one other grandchild. My brother had married an intelligent, educated, Hispanic woman named Maria, who was a middle school principal. My brother adored her, and they were very happy together. When Greyson was six years old, James and Maria had their first child, an absolutely gorgeous son named Marcos. When Greyson and I moved back to California, Marcos was two years old and my brother was a stay-at-home dad. I don't think it was their plan for my brother to stay at home, but Marcos had exhibited autistic behaviors since he was a baby, just like Greyson. For example, like Greyson, Marcos never made eye contact, never smiled, and never cried. But one behavior they didn't share was that Marcos was superhumanly strong. He was doing things like walking independently by eight months old. At age one, Marcos would climb the refrigerator using only the handles down the center. My brother would walk into the kitchen and find Marcos sitting on top of the refrigerator. Another behavior that was very different from Greyson was that Marcos didn't demonstrate any sense of fear and had an extremely high pain threshold. Since he had no fear, he often hurt himself—sometimes even bleeding profusely—but he never acknowledged that he was hurt. Greyson was the opposite—

he was so careful that by eight years old he had never even seen blood. Marcos also didn't show any signs of speaking by age two, which was a common symptom of autism that Greyson did not exhibit. But in 2002, doctors still wouldn't diagnose autism at age two. However, any parent of an autistic child can tell you they knew by this age. Unlike me, Maria and my brother recognized and accepted their son's behaviors as signs of autism. I had the actual diagnosis, but believed Greyson would become an amazing success story: "Breaking News: Autistic Man Named New CEO of Microsoft!"

I moved to California in time to apply for teaching positions —public school teaching positions because I was able to obtain an emergency teaching certificate while my official teaching certificate was being processed. I missed teaching so much and looked forward to working for someone other than Queen Linda or Frumpy. *How about a guy this time? Men are so much easier to please and aren't catty. I can't stand catty women.* I applied for every teaching position within an hour of my parents' house, and I got one interview at a middle school. One.

When I drove to the interview, which was about thirty minutes away, it became quite apparent that the neighborhood where the school was located was not so great. The streets were lined with small, old, rickety houses with front yards full of weeds, car parts, and discarded toys. But that didn't deter me at all. I drove down the poverty-stricken streets thinking, *I bet I can make a difference at this school.*

When I arrived, the principal of the middle school greeted me. *A man, thank heavens! This should be easy.* Smile, smile. Insert educational buzzword here, add an acronym there. Teaching is my jam, and so on and so forth. Fifth generation teacher here. Bada bing. Needless to say, I got the job.

I soon found out that being a middle school teacher was an entirely different beast than being an elementary school teacher. In elementary school, all the students love and want to please their teacher. In middle school, they want to fuck them up. I was given the assignment of teaching math to seventh and eighth grade ESL (English as a Second Language) students. Ha! During my interview, I must've failed to mention that the entire course of my life was altered because I failed algebra. However, since I'd earned 108 percent in my college algebra class, I felt qualified to teach math. On the other hand, I was totally not prepared to be an ESL teacher. I didn't know a lick of Spanish, and I was only provided textbooks in English. *How'd they come up with this assignment?*

A week later: *Ah, yes, I know how they came up with this assignment.* It was called "the teaching position no one else wanted," and it quickly became apparent that I'd been given the lowest-functioning, lowest-income, rough-around-the-edges group of students who hardly spoke English. *Welcome aboard, sucka!*

I was still excited to have the job, even though my students glared at me like they were planning to murder me and sell my organs. At least planning my murder required math. Ya know, time, location, average number of shots it takes to hit a moving target—stuff like that. Maybe I could take everyone's plan and compare the data in a bar graph. Ooh, or a pie chart!

Not all my students were scary as hell. Some were really sweet and told me I was their favorite teacher and that they never understood math before me. My formula for teaching math was remembering how my high school algebra teacher taught math and doing the exact opposite.

Another plus about my job was that my boss seemed relatively normal and nice. *Phew*. His name was Mr. Pierce, and he was a little man with a bit of a Napoleon complex. It was too bad I couldn't tell him I knew firsthand that height had nothing to do with penis size.

As usual, I dove into my job with the goal of perfection. I inherited the perfectionist trait from my father and the creativity trait from my mother. It's a shame that the unveiling of these traits didn't happen until adulthood. I also suffered from Post Traumatic Queen Linda Disorder (PTQLD). Symptoms included, but weren't limited to, the uncontrollable urge to: place overly detailed lesson plans on Napoleon's desk every Monday morning at eight o'clock sharp, decorate my room like nobody's business, oversee the student council, create the school's first cheerleading and dance teams, and say yes to any and all additional duties.

For my cheer team, I managed to scrounge up eight girls. There were slim pickins' at that school, and only two girls showed real potential. But we practiced and practiced and practiced every single day after school, until I ultimately transformed them into the talent equivalent of Clay Aiken. They cheered at every soccer game because that was the only sport at the school. Eventually, I signed up the girls for a cheer competition thinking it would be a good experience for them. Ironically, the girls won first place because we were, unknowingly, the only team in our division. We were so excited because it was the first trophy ever won by the school, so that was supercool. Truth be told, they would've gotten creamed had I placed them in any other division. Regardless, the girls had a great time, and that's what truly matters.

· · ·

My plan of moving Greyson across country primarily to get him out of an alternative school was working like a charm. Greyson was attending public school while I crossed my fingers, held my breath, and said my prayers. *Surely by now the school received his file via Pony Express.* Schools in California were so poor that they didn't even have fax machines in 2002. Greyson's third grade teacher was a man, and men are generally harder to rattle, so that made me hopeful. Plus, Greyson was doing better by age eight. He still had episodes, but their frequency had greatly lessened in the past couple years.

Greyson did have an episode when my parents and I took him to the mall for new clothes and shoes. As we were walking through the mall, one of Greyson's shoelaces broke, and he insisted he could no longer walk. When I asked him to try, he acted as though his legs were amputated. The more my parents and I insisted that he could, indeed, walk 150 feet to the shoe store, the more traumatic his lace-breaking incident became. He began listing all the reasons why it was impossible to continue walking in his condition. We suggested he take off his shoes and walk. Nope. We suggested he remove both laces. Nope. In desperation we suggested he crawl. Nope. I finally offered to carry him. Nope. That was it, we were stuck in that spot in the middle of the mall for the remainder of existence because *that* was what made more sense in Greyson's brain. Greyson's brilliance never set up camp at the Common Sense KOA.

After we'd waged an impossible-to-win argument for an hour, I attempted to pick up Greyson and carry him. The store was so close I could see it! At that point, he physically went out of control—screaming and thrashing about, making it impossible for me to carry him. All passersby got a great show for their judgmental enjoyment. My favorites were the ones who made disapproving sounds ("Humph!") or comments ("Idiot!") as they passed. I'm sure they all had loads of experience with children with Greyson's diagnoses.

Calming Greyson down from his episode took an additional forty-five minutes, holding us in that spot for almost two hours. I decided to convince the shoe store clerk to let me bring a few single shoes to Greyson so he could pick his favorite and try them on. I know you're thinking, *Just buy him any pair and make him live with it.* Or better yet, *He doesn't deserve new shoes anymore.* Ha! Spoken by someone with "normal" kids or no children at all. Greyson's sensory processing disorder caused him to have an oversensitivity to textures, which made it imperative for him to have comfortable shoes. That was also why Greyson never wore a pair of jeans or anything with a tag. Anything shy of a team of men with a straitjacket wouldn't get Greyson to leave that spot in the middle of the mall. So it was either that or find new shoes that Greyson approved.

After I made a few trips back and forth between the shoe store and Greyson, toting several solitary shoes for Greyson to inspect and try on, he picked a pair he liked, and we went on with our day as if the incident never happened. Every time an episode ended, Greyson recovered in a snap, but I did not. His episodes left me pondering, *What the hell was that?*

By October 2002, Greyson and I had been in California almost four months, and I was finally beginning to feel acclimated. Greyson hadn't been kicked out of school yet, and my job was going really well. I'd already had one formal observation (a nerve-racking experience during which principals scrutinize the delivery of a lesson) and had earned a wonderful review from my principal. The superintendent, who popped into my classroom periodically, even complimented my teaching. Both were also pleased with my extensive work with the cheerleaders.

Just when I was beginning to no longer think about Michael, he decided to give me a call completely out of the blue. I was on my way home from work when my cell phone —a state-of-the-art flip phone—rang.

"How are you?" he whispered.

"I'm fabulous." *Kinda.* "You?" *I actually don't care.*

"I'm okay. I miss you."

"I miss you too." *Shit, that slipped.*

Ten minutes of awkward small talk.

"Can I visit you?" he asked.

Silence.

"So . . . can I?" he repeated.

"Why? What's the point?"

"I miss you."

"If you buy a ticket, rent a car, and get a hotel, I'll find time to see you," I said acting all tough.

"K," he mumbled.

"Let me know when you have it all figured out." *I am Claire, hear me roar! Stupid, stupid, stupid Claire.*

I had a hard time believing Michael would make all the arrangements to see me because such grand gestures just weren't his thing. But a week later, there he was on my parents' doorstep. *Crap, you're still hot.* He grabbed me and held me tight in a way I don't remember him ever doing in Chicago. "You have no idea how much I've missed you."

"Ready? Let's go," attempting to brush off his affection.

Insert superfun date here. The kind of date where we held hands, walked with a spring in our step, giggled nonstop, and fed each other perfectly assembled bites during dinner. The kind of date where people watched us and then got mad at their significant other for no reason.

"When can I come back?" he asked.

"When you buy a ticket, rent a car, and get a hotel again." I refused to put in any effort when four months earlier, I was front and center, ready to get married. He's the one that screwed up, not me.

"I'll see you in two weeks."

"K." *Yeah, right,* I thought. *Like you're going to do all this again in two weeks.*

But two weeks later, there he was on my parents' doorstep. And, once again, there we were having a great time like a couple of lovebirds. *I'm way too forgiving and cool.*

After that, we started talking on the phone every night for hours after Greyson went to bed. Then, like clockwork, he came to visit every two weeks, planning and paying for everything. He didn't do that in Chicago. Back then, he had no qualms about us taking turns picking up the check. He had a tendency to treat me like his buddy—not his woman— which I never liked. Maybe before he thought he was a hot commodity. Now, he was groveling, and I kinda liked it.

Months went by and all was well with Michael, with my job, and with Greyson, who was miraculously still at the public school. I think it helped that his teacher had the personality of a brick and didn't seem to care about anything. Word on the street was that his teacher was a putz. *I'll take it!*

I loved my job so much that in January 2003, during my second semester there, I started the school's first-ever dance team. Yeah, I know, I'm a show-off. I have a go-big-or-go-home attitude that I believe has served me well as a teacher. The students embraced the dance team much more than they did the cheer team, so I didn't have to scrounge for girls—I got twenty-five girls to sign up without even trying! Perhaps it was because by then, I'd proved myself as a teacher and cheer coach. Dance was more fun than cheer for me. I choreographed awesome dances, if I do say so myself. All my years in cheer and dance really came in handy.

Michael continued to surprise me. Without fail, he appeared on my parents' doorstep every other Friday night. And, without fail, I never planned anything or picked up the check. It was my new definition of fun. Michael also had to entertain himself during the days he was in town because I refused to let him interfere with my time with Greyson. Michael never dared to complain because he knew he'd done this to himself. It seemed like before he came crawling back to me (as I like to put it), Michael had attended Learn How to Become a Gentleman camp.

Although one particular weekend, he screwed up. In 2003, Valentine's Day landed on a Friday, but he'd visited the Friday before, which meant we'd miss Valentine's Day together. I thought that was poor planning on his part. In my mind, he should've just skipped visiting the previous weekend.

When Valentine's Day arrived, I came home from school balancing a stack of schoolwork in my arms that came up to my chin. (Queen Linda would've been SO proud.) I always got caught up on grading and planning during weekend nights when Michael wasn't in town. As I carefully balanced all my work on my parents' countertop, I noticed a huge bouquet of flowers. *Aw . . . Michael sent flowers. That's a first. Although I'm not much of a flower person. Seems like such a waste of money. They're beautiful and all, but I'd prefer a new pair of shoes in that vase.*

I approached the flowers and read the card. "Get packed. Your chariot arrives in an hour."

I looked up and my parents were standing there— clenching their fists, smiling from ear to ear, bopping up and down like Kelly Clarkson, and squealing with delight.

No way! No WAY!

My brain was going a million miles an hour. Michael had e-mailed me from work just two hours earlier. How could he possibly be here? I talked to him on my way home from work, and he was acting totally normal—like he was just hanging out on the couch at home. That stinker. He was a way better liar than I realized, but other than that, I was superexcited.

"What are you waiting for?!" My parents couldn't control their excitement. They're so cute.

"What?"

"Pack!"

Oh yeah . . . I need to pack.

I packed a suitcase for a weekend away. I had never been away from Greyson for a weekend, or even a full day, so the thought of it was strange, yet exciting. An adult weekend . . . with adults doing adulty things.

An hour later, a beautiful, white, stretch limo showed up at my parents' house. *Nice work Mikey.* The chauffeur immediately took my suitcase, and I got inside assuming Michael would be there. But he wasn't. Instead of Michael, there were trays of food sprawled all over the limo. Fair trade. Beautiful trays of berries and melons, veggies and dips, cookies and cakes. *Yes, food, I love you too.*

The chauffeur drove and drove and wouldn't spill the beans on where we were going. If I didn't have food keeping me busy, I would've pressed the issue a little more. I can be very persuasive when my mouth's not full.

The limo finally pulled up to a secluded beach. The beach

was so beautiful, and the sun was just beginning to set. I scoped the horizon and saw a man off in the distance. That must be Michael! I ran to him and kissed his gorgeous full lips. He had a picnic set up with a blanket, a picnic basket, and a bottle of wine. He knew eating trays of food during the past hour had only gotten me warmed up.

He looked into my eyes with a strange look that was unfamiliar to me. Love? Devotion? Fear? He proceeded to get down on one knee and asked me to marry him and asked to be a father to Greyson.

I screamed, "Yes!" My hands were shaking as he put a stunning, two-carat solitaire, platinum ring on my finger. I didn't need to think about my answer that time.

We laid on the blanket, enjoyed the sunset, fed each other cheese and crackers, and drank wine. Michael told me that he'd timed his proposal so it would be during the sunset. *Where has this Michael been hiding?*

After the sunset, we continued our evening at a fancy steak restaurant because no matter how much I've eaten, I always have room for steak. Over dinner, Michael told me that he'd booked a room at a resort for the weekend, officially earning him a rock-solid A+ in the wedding proposal department.

Four months later, the day after my last day of teaching, about forty-five of our closest friends and relatives gathered for our wedding. Picture white seats, a white walkway, and a breathtaking ocean view on the mountaintop of Mount Soledad in La Jolla, California. My aunt, who's a minister, performed the ceremony and did a great job making it profound. My wedding dress was off-the-rack from Saks Fifth Avenue. Actually, it wasn't a wedding dress. It was an elegant, classy yet sexy, ivory dress, and I totally loved it. It was very Caroline Kennedy.

Our reception was on a deck right on the ocean at a

beautiful French restaurant in La Jolla. My parents, Michael, and I had checked out a few other locations, but when we took one look at that deck all four of us said, "This is it." We served multiple flavors of cheesecake instead of wedding cake because I've never tasted a good wedding cake. We had my favorite pineapple champagne from a local winery for the toast. The food was insanely delicious because delicious food was as important as a delicious groom. The open bar consisted of anything the heart desired—from drinks with fancy fruit garnishes and sugar rims to drinks with Baileys and little chocolate shavings. I planned the wedding and reception in about two weeks. Easy-peasy. I'd never had the desire for a traditional wedding—long ceremony, banquet hall reception, choice of mediocre chicken or steak, and a deejay playing songs off a list called "What to Play at Every Wedding Reception in the Universe." My wedding was simple, sophisticated, and scrumptious. And I wouldn't change a thing.

NAGNESS

2003–2004

*R*ight before we'd broken up a year earlier, Michael had bought a brand-new house. I'd helped him pick out all the colors and upgrades, so it had felt like my house too. Needless to say, Greyson and I moved back to Chicago since Michael had the better paying job and the brand-new house. Plus, Greyson had survived an entire school year in California without getting kicked out, so I figured that the Chicago schools had to give him another chance.

The school year in California ended much later than the school year in Chicago. Michael and I also went on a ten-day cruise to Alaska for our honeymoon. Can you believe I had ten whole days of adulting? By the time we finally made the move back to Chicago, it was almost time for the school year to start. I quickly applied for some teaching positions at nearby Catholic schools since I didn't have an Illinois certificate yet, and Illinois didn't offer emergency certificates like California did. Catholic schools accept out-of-state certificates; public schools do not.

I was called for three interviews and was offered all three positions. I picked the one that was ten minutes from our house, which also happened to be the grade level I was most excited about: second grade. Plus, the Catholic school was 99 percent Hispanic, and after loving my position in California, I felt a connection with the Hispanic culture.

My new principal was an elderly former nun named Agnes. *I wonder what happened? How does someone become a former nun except in the movies?* My guess was that she got horny because she actually had a boyfriend. A boyfriend! Yet, Agnes was still a bit crabby. Maybe she realized penises are overrated. She'd left the convent when all she really needed was a vibrator.

Every morning, I got to work exactly on time—never one minute late and usually a few minutes early. Yet, every morning when I walked in, she tapped her watch and gave me a stern look as if to say, "Cutting it a little close, aren't ya?" Teachers were asked to arrive thirty minutes before the students. *That's when I arrive, so what's the problem? I need to talk to that boyfriend of hers and tell him to up his game—remind him that she chose his penis over the Lord.*

Agnes (actually Nagness seems more accurate) also insisted on typed, detailed lesson plans on her desk every Monday morning. *Ha, that's a snack, sister!* At our monthly staff meetings, she used my lesson plans as a visual aid to show all the other teachers what lesson plans should look like. I'm sure everyone loved that. I could tell Nagness liked me but didn't want to show it. Her face would probably crack if she smiled. She was, however, cool in one respect— she served wine at our staff meetings. Wine! I love Catholics.

Being at a new school, I couldn't stop at just having the cutest classroom and the best lesson plans, I had to start the school's first dance team as well. We practiced twice a week and performed at school assemblies since the school didn't have any sports. They actually didn't have assemblies either, I created those too. For the assemblies, I made up funny skits for willing teachers to perform. Skits that often involved teachers dancing and telling jokes—the students thought it was hilarious. Even Nagness had a hard time keeping a straight face.

The school year was going great for Greyson as well. And by great, I mean Greyson hadn't been kicked out yet, which was my normal measurement for how a school year was going. I had successfully enrolled Greyson at a traditional public school. We just went to enrollment wearing trench coats, big sunglasses, and our hair dyed black. *I'm kidding, black hair doesn't go with my skin tone.* But I may have forgotten to mention some minor details like Greyson's diagnoses and that he'd attended an alternative school in the past, yada yada yada. Basically, I beat the system by just moving across the country. Twice. No biggie. And I did have a new last name, so that worked well with my plan.

Greyson's new last name was also in the works. We'd hired a lawyer and started the adoption process to satisfy my marriage stipulations. Yes, I realize I was forcing Michael to adopt Greyson, but he hadn't said a word opposing it since he knew I wouldn't marry him otherwise. Actually, Michael was really trying to bond with Greyson. Once a week, he took Greyson to a nearby ice cream shop with tables that doubled as chessboards. They would go there—just the two of them—and have ice cream and play chess. Michael was very proud that he was crowned "chess champion" when he was a child. He attempted to use his decades-old title to jokingly talk smack with Greyson, but Greyson didn't understand teasing, so he'd respond with a stop-trying-to-amuse-me look.

At the time, Greyson also played the violin. He wouldn't play sports or do anything physical, but he showed an interest in music. He chose the violin, and I couldn't decide whether that was impressive or bizarre for a nine-year-old with no musical background. Another boy in the neighborhood played the trombone in the same orchestra, so his mother and I set up a carpool system since they had practice so frequently. At least that was her reason. My reason was a desperate attempt to find Greyson his first friend. Carpooling went okay for about a month, then the mother called me and said she could no longer drive Greyson. When I asked why, she said, and I quote, "I don't like your son." I can't make this shit up. She literally said that. At least she was honest. In Oklahoma, no one would say such a thing. But in Chicago, people cut the crap. I do prefer that approach over the born-again Christians who offer up their best fake smiles, cheerful voices, and pretend niceness before slowly exiling you from their inner circle of perfection.

Greyson was doing very well academically. He had never received a grade lower than an A. When he got straight As at the alternative school, I thought, *Big deal*. Then, in California, his teacher was so lackadaisical that again I thought, *Big deal*. But by this time, Greyson had a really great teacher and his report card still sported straight As. It would've been a perfect report card if I'd stopped reading after the "Academic Grades" section. But when I continued scrolling down to the "Life Skills" section, there were dreaded check marks instead of perfect pluses after every social and behavioral statement.

"Solves problems appropriately." Big check.

"Observes classroom rules." Big ole check.

"Exhibits respectful behavior." Check, check, check.

Okay, so maybe Greyson was still struggling behaviorally,

but at least he wasn't pummeling the crap out of anyone—or at least I didn't think he was. They didn't have a box for that in the Life Skills section of the report card. I was still superproud of him. He was at a traditional school and was getting straight As! That's my boy!

*B*y 2004, I was in my second year at the Catholic school. I loved my job, but public school teachers made at least double my salary. I had to stay an additional year because guess how long it took Illinois to approve an out-of-state teaching certificate? Thirteen months. Yep, government turnaround at its finest. No, I wasn't short any classes or deficient in any way; it just literally took thirteen months to get a sheet of paper. God bless America.

That year, a new teacher named Molly was hired to teach kindergarten at my school. She was super-duper annoying. She was all, "I'm the greatest teacher in the world with all my darling projects and creative ideas." She was also really cute and thin. Ugh. And she talked way too loud. Plus, she always wanted to help me with the assemblies and had all these annoyingly brilliant ideas. It was so exasperating.

Or—and I'm just throwing this out there—maybe she was the only teacher I ever worked with that shared my perfectionism and enthusiasm. *Am I that annoying? Do I talk that loud?* I do think I was a smidge cuter and a tad thinner. Ha!

I found myself writing down her ideas behind her back just in case I ever taught kindergarten. My second grade ideas were better—or maybe equally as adorable. Nah, mine were better.

A couple months into the school year, Nagness picked Molly and me to go to a training seminar about an hour and a half away. She suggested we carpool since it was such a far distance. *Seriously? Why did you have to suggest that right in front of Molly? I'd rather drive in peace than listen to her shrieky voice for three hours.*

At the next staff meeting, Molly verbalized everything that we'd learned in training. Vomit. Furthermore, Nagness showed both my lesson plans *and* Molly's lesson plans to the staff. *Wait a second, it's my job to piss off the staff, not hers.* I smirked when I noticed mine were three pages typed and hers were only two.

In the fall of 2004, Greyson's adoption was finalized. We celebrated at Greyson's favorite restaurant. I was ecstatic about the adoption, but Greyson could take it or leave it. He still never showed emotion—never cried, never smiled, never laughed, never seemed . . . happy. He was like a robot, my sweet little robot—except when he'd have an episode. I guess he had two states of mind—nothingness and scary as hell. *Is scary as hell an emotion?*

Thankfully, by this time, Greyson's episodes had almost completely disappeared. It was probably due to a combination of Greyson getting older and me knowing what subjects to skirt around. He was still by no means an easy child. He'd argue if I said the sky was blue when really it was bluish-green. I'd still occasionally lock our bedroom door at night when, for instance, he glared at me for an hour because I'd made tacos for dinner, which was not on the short list of things Greyson enjoyed eating. I now had to consider what Michael liked too.

Greyson still hadn't made a friend or been invited to a party, even though I continued to throw lavish birthday and Halloween parties every year and invited everyone in his class. You would think at some point another mom would say, "Hey Joey, how about inviting that Greyson kid since you went to his party?" But no. Apparently, word had spread that Greyson was the naughty boy at school. That didn't deter moms from dropping their kids off at Greyson's parties while they grabbed Starbucks with friends. *What do I have to do to get my kid invited to a birthday party? Or a playdate?*

I sent Greyson to school with little playdate cards with my number and e-mail address on them in his backpack. They were like business cards, but for playdates. I saw them on Etsy and thought they were cute. Surely playdate cards would equal playdates. I thought Greyson had a better chance of just handing someone a card versus trying to interact with them. Then their mother would see the card and say, "Oh, how cute, a playdate card, let me just dial this number and set up a playdate." I may have had a glass of wine while I was perusing Etsy that night. I told Greyson if he ever played with anyone—anyone at all—he should give them his card and invite them over. Those cards never moved.

There weren't many kids in our neighborhood to socialize with either—just a small handful that included trombone boy whose mother didn't like Greyson. I'm sure she'd let everyone know Greyson was the naughty boy on the street. I'd noticed that when the few kids played in the neighborhood, it was on the opposite end of the street, a block away from our house. I wondered if that was intentional.

Greyson had no friends. I had no friends. I'd landed a husband but remained friendless for over a decade. Anna got sick and Rachel got married shortly after Greyson was born. All my other friends dropped like flies when Greyson was conceived. Then I went down that illusory born-again Christian path, desperately seeking friends—or maybe a drop of support. *It's so funny how I thought born-again Christians were actually Christians. I crack myself up.* Then I learned that moms avoid moms of naughty kids and that kids play on the opposite end of the street. Making friends as a teacher was also difficult. Teachers spend their days within the four walls of their classrooms, which is not conducive for socialization. My twenty-minute lunch period was typically spent inhaling a sandwich while prepping for an after-lunch lesson, so that didn't help me make any friends.

I wished Rachel and I were still close. But by that time, her second child was on the way. Her first daughter was flawless. Indubitably. When she was a baby, she giggled, she slept, she nursed, she made eye contact. I sometimes asked Rachel if Greyson and I could go to her family's cottage in Lake Geneva for a weekend. But after she got married, she said their cottage was too packed with family. I later found out that she'd invited other friends. Friends with perfect children to play with her perfect children. I felt crushed, and our lifelong friendship fizzled to maybe dinner every six months. When we were together, we laughed so hysterically that tears rolled down our bright red faces. We were always the last people to leave the restaurant at night, and it made me wonder why she didn't want me anymore.

Greyson was in his second year at a public school and still hadn't been kicked out. He continued to get straight As without ever once doing homework. I thought the no homework thing would change since, at this point, Greyson was in fifth grade. Yet he never brought home a single page of homework. In kindergarten, I just figured, *Well, it is kindergarten.* At the alternative school, I was like, *Well, it is an alternative school*. But by this time, he was at a great school with great teachers. Every time I asked Greyson if he had homework, he'd say that he'd finished it at school, and yet he still continued to bring home straight A report cards. Apparently, schoolwork came easily for Greyson. I beamed with pride when I got his report cards. I wanted to slip a copy to all the moms who gave us the cold shoulder with a note that said, "Take that bitches!" Of course, I'd have to exclude the Life Skills section.

With the end of the school year fast approaching, I applied at every district within an hour of my house since I finally had my Illinois certification. I received one call from a district that was exactly an hour away. I had to schedule my interview after school because Nagness didn't allow sick days. In two years, I'd taken one sick day, well, half a sick day. Nagness finally let me go home when she found me on the bathroom floor, sobbing and sweating from the flu while the secretary watched my class. The day before, I had told Nagness that I was feeling sick, but she'd said, "Don't even think about taking a sick day," even though I got seven sick days per year according to my contract. I'm pretty sure that was illegal. Catholic schools paid so poorly that it was difficult to get a sub. Catholic schools paid subs a meager fifty dollars per day, while public schools paid them over a hundred dollars per day. So it was a huge inconvenience for Nagness when a teacher was out because she'd have a hard time getting a sub. Molly also came to work sick one day. She ran out of her classroom and threw up in the bathroom. That was Molly's only sick day—I mean half sick day.

When I showed up for my interview, I went into the principal's office and the two of us talked for about an hour. The interview was very laid-back, very casual, and the best part: the principal was a man! *Yay!* He seemed very nice too —very soft spoken, kind eyes, well dressed. His name was Tim. *I like Tim.*

A few days after my interview, I received a call from the district. Tim wanted a second interview. *A second one? An hour wasn't enough?* I set up another interview, again, after school.

I showed up for my second interview and was sent down a quiet hallway to another room. When I opened the door, there was a large rectangular table surrounded by women with enormous smiles. I figured they were all teachers, so I couldn't believe they were willing to stay at work so late. But then I remembered they weren't making $28,000 per year. Soon, my heart started pounding, and I felt sick to my stomach. The room was chalky white with standard cheap fluorescent lighting. One of the lights was faintly flickering. *Ah, this must be where they hold their IEP meetings.* I mustered up a big, fake smile and said, "Hi! My name is Claire!" *I've got this.*

The interview went on for an hour . . . or maybe twelve, I'm not sure. They used a round-robin approach, each one of them firing questions at me like a police interrogation. As I answered, they all smiled, took notes, and nodded as if in agreement. I preferred my last interview with just Tim. *Maybe I should've brought muffins.*

A few days later, I got another call from the district. They wanted me to come in and teach a lesson. *Seriously?* I couldn't take a day off work unless I made myself vomit. I explained again that I couldn't come during school hours and asked if I could videotape myself teaching in my classroom. They agreed, so I made a videotape of myself teaching, mailed it, and waited.

A week later, a woman from the district contacted me and explained that Nagness hadn't returned her calls to check my reference. I told her that I imagined my principal was not happy to see me go. Without me, there wouldn't be a dance team or assemblies. (Although I'm sure Molly would never let that happen. Unless, I thought with a smile, dancing was the one thing Molly couldn't do.) The woman from the district told me she'd talk to Tim and get back to me.

You've got to be kidding me, Nagness. You're going to hold me hostage at your school?

Meanwhile, I was making small talk with Molly in the hallway after school. She told me she'd applied for other teaching jobs as well. We were both stressed out and had no one else to talk to since all the other teachers left at three. She told me she'd had an interview to teach in China. She looked really upset and unexpectedly pulled me into my classroom like we were best friends and she couldn't wait to tell me her secret. But since we weren't friends, I was caught off guard. She started tearing up and said Nagness was refusing to e-mail a letter of recommendation to the company that hired teachers to go to China. She said they'd asked Nagness twice, but didn't get a response. I looked at her and said, "Oh my gosh! She's doing the exact same thing to me! I have another job offer, but she's not returning their calls for a reference!"

That very moment in time marked the moment I made my new best friend. Molly and I sat in my classroom and bitched about Nagness. We laughed about our half sick days, our competitive lesson plans, and that we'd be teaching there until we were eighty-five because we'd be too poor to retire and could never get a reference. We agreed that Nagness needed more sex. *Molly's voice wasn't so shrieky after all,* I thought.

A couple days later, we both got word that we'd been offered our new jobs, despite Nagness's interference. So Molly was leaving for China. *Total buzzkill.* We'd missed out on a whole year of friendship, and now she was leaving for the other side of the planet—literally.

Molly ended the school year with an amazing kindergarten show for parents and the whole school. It was almost as impressive as my dancers. Almost. *Who am I kidding? It was adorable.* I asked Molly if I could have a copy of the poem she wrote and read intermittently throughout the show. It was ingenious. She happily gave it to me, and I added it to my secret Molly file. The file I thought I'd never use was now going to come in very handy because the new job I was offered was for kindergarten! *Yippee!*

MIDDLE SCHOOL AND A MASTER'S DEGREE

2005–2008

I'd say the following years were my favorite with Greyson. I always knew Greyson was special, that he was put on this planet to make a difference. I firmly believed that God would never waste such an amazing mind on someone who wasn't here for a very important reason. Greyson may have lacked social skills, but there are so many great people in history with similar stories. Greyson's social awkwardness was one of the things that made him unique. His literal mind was so real, so raw; it was as if not being able to interact with others helped his mind remain untainted. Things most people did solely because it was considered acceptable, polite, popular, or normal, Greyson deemed illogical, unwarranted, meaningless, and wasteful. When he verbalized his puzzlement of certain social norms, I was always like, "Yeah, that makes perfect sense," and it made me love his brain even more. He intrigued me and made me look at things like no one else did. His brain was untraditional in a wonderful, fascinating way. I felt like the luckiest mom in the world. Anyone could raise an easy, normal child. That almost sounded mundane. Few moms were so blessed to witness firsthand the progression of a genius mind at every stage of development. Greyson made life challenging yet interesting, and I wouldn't trade him for any other child. I prayed to God every night and thanked Him for choosing me to raise such a remarkable son. I was giddy with excitement to see what the future held for Greyson.

Greyson's sixth grade year was equally academically successful. He astonished me with his continuation of straight A report cards while maintaining a 0 percent homework rate. I stopped reading the Life Skills section and accepted that Greyson didn't fit into the Life Skills mold. At the end of sixth grade, Greyson was presented with the President's Award for Educational Excellence—an academic award that recognizes a student's academic success when graduating from elementary, middle, or high school. I also found out from Greyson's teacher that he'd been recommended for the middle school's gifted program as a result of his grades and standardized test scores. I always giggled when I saw results from Greyson's standardized tests because he always scored in the ninety-ninth percentile in every single subject. Greyson later accepted the invitation into the highly respected, sought-after, gifted program.

Greyson continued his academic success in the gifted program during middle school. The teachers were fantastic and really challenged him. Greyson, however, could no longer maintain his 0 percent homework policy. Teachers gave an astronomical amount of homework, which he reluctantly completed each night despite the fact that he referred to it as an "exorbitant waste of his time." Greyson understood the material without all the extra practice, therefore, he found homework a superfluous activity. Homework was forcing him to surrender to society's obtuse conventions, which was very un-Greyson-like. It went against every fiber of Greyson's oppositional-defiant-disorder being.

Greyson and I had been inseparable from the day he was born and always shared a close relationship. We spent every free moment together. Since Greyson didn't have friends, he willingly spent every free moment he had with me. But I worried that he wouldn't want to spend time with me when he became a teenager. Clearly, I wanted him to have friends (more than anything in the world, really), but I wondered if he'd be like most teenagers and not want to be around me anymore. We usually did something fun every weekend during the school year. Then we spent our summers going to water parks, movies, museums, parks, festivals, and the beach. I loved being a teacher and having summers off to spend with him. Every summer Michael moaned and groaned, wishing he'd chosen my profession. I teased Michael every day as Greyson and I headed out the door for our daily adventure.

Greyson and I also did an insane amount of fun things around the holidays. Greyson's favorite holiday was Halloween, so we'd have a great time together every October. Every year, we'd frequent several pumpkin patches and haunted hayrides. We did something Halloween–related every weekend throughout October.

From the time Greyson was eight years old, I'd thrown big Halloween parties and invited his entire class because, apparently, the lack of reciprocation from birthday parties just wasn't enough. My thinking was that Greyson would never be invited to parties, so I had to bring the parties to him. Every year, we'd decorate the front yard together and turn the basement into a haunted house. We wallpapered the walls with large, black plastic bags, hung several from ceiling to floor to make a maze, and then filled it with scary decorations. At the end of the maze, we left an open space where we set up Halloween games like ghost darts, Bozo buckets with cauldrons, and a ring toss using witch hats. (I had a ridiculous amount of decorations because every year after Halloween, we went crazy buying decorations on clearance.) I made Halloween–themed food like green Jell-O made with a brain mold, cupcakes with gummy worms, powdered donut eyeballs—gross stuff like that. I always came up with a creative scavenger hunt too. The kids split into teams and had to hunt for items throughout the neighborhood. Some years, I turned the scavenger hunt into a murder mystery to solve from clues they collected.

Those were my favorite memories with Greyson. I was convinced the more love, effort, energy, and time I gave Greyson, the more likely he'd succeed in life. Since the day Greyson was born, I felt like my sole purpose was to prepare him for his bright future. I thought showering him with unconditional love and creating positive life experiences was all he needed. He had the brains, he had the looks, he had the loving family, all I had to do was pave his way with wonderful memories and experiences. That's a surefire formula for raising a successful and confident adult, right? Of course, it is!

As smart as Greyson was and as much as I tried and tried and tried to continue a close relationship with him, his favorite pastimes were: arguing with me, questioning every word I said, refusing to comply with requests regardless of simplicity, blaming me for his mistakes, and deliberately upsetting me.

And all just for fun!

Not to worry, Greyson spread his love and cheer to those all around—Michael, his teachers, his peers, the employees at Chipotle. He did not discriminate. We all got to partake in the joys of Greyson's oppositional defiant disorder.

In spite of his sparkling personality, at the end of middle

school, Greyson was recommended for a gifted program at one of the high schools in our district. It was even more difficult to get accepted into this program because only sixty students were accepted out of the district's thirty-nine thousand. To get into the program, the students had to be recommended by a teacher, their standardized and gifted test scores had to be above the ninety-fifth percentile, and they had to pass an interview process. *Uh-oh.* Well, the first two requirements were easy-peasy, lemon-squeezy (sorry, sometimes my annoying kindergarten teacher voice slips out).

Three weeks after his interview, we received a rejection letter. I called the director of the program and asked for a clarification as to why Greyson wasn't accepted. He told me exactly what I already knew, "Greyson's scores are off the charts, but his interview went very poorly." I thanked him and briefly explained the social struggles Greyson has had since he was little. "I see," he responded, as if I just wasted ninety seconds of his life.

A week later I received a second letter. "After further consideration, Greyson has been accepted into the gifted program."

Huh?

When I told Greyson, he . . . smiled. It was a bit mechanical, but he did it. He actually smiled! Just thinking about it makes me smile. So the following school year, Greyson started high school in a gifted program so advanced that with successful completion of the program, he could start college as a junior. There was a possibility that he could actually graduate college at age nineteen. Nice! Not to mention it would save us a ton of money on college tuition.

. . .

During this time, I hit the ground running with my kindergarten teaching position. Being the only kindergarten teacher at the school gave me the freedom to do whatever my heart desired. I started the school's first dance team, arranged multiple classroom events throughout the year, and organized an adorable end-of-the-year show (secret Molly file, *shhh*). We had a ton of fun, and I was also recognized for drastically increasing kindergarten reading scores.

I loved my principal as much as I had my principal in Minnesota. He was so nice, so calm, so sweet, and stayed so out of my way. He trusted me and my abilities, which made me work even harder. Unfortunately, he left at the end of my third year. He put a personal note on my desk before he left that made me cry. I still have it to this day. When he interviewed for his new principalship in another district, he chose me as a reference, and I was interviewed regarding his performance as a principal. I felt honored that he trusted me with this very important task.

I also loved the superintendent. My classroom was located in what most would call "the worst location in the world." It was directly across from the superintendent's office, so he popped his head into my classroom regularly, and we often ran into each other in the hallway. He was not a well-liked man in the district. In an effort to make changes in the district, he'd fired several teachers. I didn't personally know the teachers he'd fired because they were at different schools, so I wasn't sure if it was warranted or not. But he was always kind to me, so I gave him the benefit of the doubt. He was also very witty. When he spoke at our district-wide professional development meetings, he'd throw in a lot of jokes, and I thought he was hilarious. Other teachers tried not to laugh. Not me. He cracked me up. Teachers always complained about him in the lunchroom. I'd just sit there and bite my tongue. I really wish I'd had this tongue-biting skill when I was in high school.

In my district, teachers were not given tenure until their fifth year, so achieving tenure was not an easy task. Every year during my first four years, teachers were always pink-slipped or laid off. Then, after the district got its numbers for the following year, those teachers would usually be rehired. The only reason I knew this was from the talk in the lunchroom. Can you believe we got a full forty minutes for lunch? I love public schools! Every year, the newer teachers would be upset, typically in tears, when they were given their pink slips. I would just sit there and listen, and over the years, I finally realized I was the only new teacher who never got pink-slipped. One day the superintendent stopped me in the hallway and said, "Every time I see you in the hallway, you're smiling. And every time I look in your classroom, you're having so much fun with the students. Thank you." That made my day . . . my week . . . my year!

Now that I had my dream job, I'd decided to go back to school to earn a master's degree. As a teacher, this is how you give yourself a huge bump in pay. I was already making double what I'd made at my previous Catholic and Christian schools, and with completion of a master's degree, my salary would go up another ten thousand dollars. Michael and I had been talking about having children of our own, but my goal was to earn my master's degree before having more children. Going to class in the evenings and doing schoolwork was not something I wanted to do with a baby.

The master's degree program took two years to complete, but it wasn't nearly as torturous as I'd anticipated. It was a ton of work, but I sat with the same three amazing women every single class for two solid years. We got along famously, and they actually made class fun. Classes were one night a week and four hours long, so we always got a dinner break.

The four of us had dinner together every class, so it was like a built-in girls' night out once a week. I actually felt like I had somewhat of a social life and had finally made some new friends. The four of us ended up graduating with straight As and continued to have dinner together once a month for many years after.

My friendship with Molly also remained intact. Although Molly had moved to China, she came to visit three times a year. I spent a lot of time with her during her visits. It was like we'd been best friends forever. I actually spent far more time with Molly who lived seven thousand miles away than I did with Rachel who lived seven miles away. Humph, it's sad really . . . the Rachel part.

Molly put effort into friendships like me. We were like Taylor Swift meets Taylor Swift. Molly was superloyal and real. It's virtually impossible to find a friend as awesome as Molly, so I'm glad we connected before she went off to China. Not only that, but she brought me awesome stuff from China like knockoff Prada bags—good ones—and actual real pearls. It was a nice bestie perk.

Molly went to China for three whole years then moved back to Chicago. While she was in China, she met her husband. Every time I tell people that, the first thing they ask is if he's Chinese, so I'll just tell you he's not. He's from Iowa and as white as a sheep. He graduated from Harvard with a degree in Mandarin and folklore. Then he went to teach in China where he met Molly. Can you believe Harvard offers a degree in Mandarin and folklore? He's like the world's smartest wizard. He's also smart because he landed Molly. She's the best.

Husband. Check.

Greyson doing well-ish. Check.

Best friend. Check.

Social life. Check.

Amazing job. Check.
Master's degree. Check.
Good income. Check.
Baby-making time!
Sounds fun, right?
Meh.

HAPPY FUCKING PRESIDENTS' DAY!

2008

*H*aving sex left and right trying to make a baby was fun the first few months, but then I was like, "Why am I not getting pregnant?" I got impregnated by Sperm Donor after a single mishap, while kinda sorta on my period, let me just reiterate. *Yuck, probably shouldn't have reminded you. It was the last day. Still gross, I know. Made me cringe too.*

Month one. No baby.

Month two. No baby.

Month three. No baby.

Month . . . ten. Still no baby.

Well, this is depressing. It's not from lack of trying either because I'm all over Michael. Hmm. . . .

On Sunday night, the night before Presidents' Day 2008, Michael and I went to his buddy's house to play poker since we had Monday off work. He's got a million friends. He's known them all since preschool, and they've stuck together all these years. They're all good guys. Nice wives too. All-American nice families with 2.5 children.

As usual, I was creaming everyone in poker. I actually

don't remember who was winning, but I'm sure it was me. It was about one o'clock in the morning, and I had to use the bathroom. Plus, I thought it'd be nice to give other people a chance to win a hand. Then the strangest thing happened in the bathroom. I pulled down my pants, and all of a sudden, *whoosh!* What seemed like a gallon of blood just spewed out of my vagina. As if a tiny and annoying being crawled into my vagina, filled a whole bucket with blood, and then dumped it in the toilet right as I began to sit. *Splash!* Blood covered the toilet. The weirdest part was that I wasn't on my period, and I felt perfectly fine. No cramping, no nausea, no nothing. (Justifiable double negative for emphasis.)

I painstakingly cleaned the bathroom after what looked like a crime scene, then returned to our poker game with what I'm sure was a confused look on my face.

"Everything okay?" they asked.

"Yeah, fine." *I think. Either that or I'm dying . . . I'm not totally sure.*

I finally pulled one of the wives aside and told her what had happened. "You should go to the emergency room," she said. *Maybe I should tell someone else. Clearly, you're no use to me.*

"I'm not bleeding anymore. I'm fine." I mean, it was only like one bucket of blood, not two. Now if there were two buckets involved, *that* would mean trouble.

I called my cousin who's a doctor. "You have to go to the emergency room. *NOW!*" she ordered.

Of course, she's going to say that. She's a doctor, and all doctors want you to go to the emergency room so they can send you lots of bills.

I should preface this by telling you that I hate doctors—not my cousin, of course, just every other doctor in existence. And according to a study by Johns Hopkins, medical mistakes are one of the leading causes of death in the

United States. Case in point: My brother almost had his leg mistakenly amputated. My uncle had to have a kidney removed after another patient's urine test results were confused with his. And my dad is partially blind in one eye—all because of dumb doctors. My father has also had two failed surgeries for his hearing at Mayo Clinic. One was because they tested the wrong ear! Needless to say, I come from a long line of doctor haters.

So it should come as no surprise that I was thinking to myself: *It's late, and I just want to go to bed. I'll go to the hospital in the morning if the blood comes back. Solid plan.*

Well, off to the hospital we went. Not sure why I changed my mind. When I told the chick at the front desk what had happened, she immediately sent me back to a room. *Interesting,* I thought. *What about the other thirty-two people in the waiting room? I'll have to remember what I told her for future emergency room visits.*

A woman who looked thrilled to be there entered my room and asked me some questions.

"Are you pregnant?"

"No."

"Have your periods been regular?"

"Yes."

"Tell me what happened."

"Bucket of blood went *whoosh* out of my vagina. That's it."

"Any pain?"

"Nope."

"Cramps?"

"Nope."

"Nausea?"

"Nope."

"Dizziness?"

"Nope."

"Light-headedness?"

"Nope." *Pretty sure that's the same thing as dizzy.*

"Diarrhea?"

Gross, no, like I'd tell you. "Nope."

"Vomiting?"

"Nope."

"Bowel pain?"

"Nope."

"Any additional bleeding after the (insert nauseating look) *'whoosh'*?"

"Nope." *Have I mentioned you're annoying? And you smell like peroxide.*

"Any other symptoms you can think of at all?"

"Nope. I feel perfect."

Annoying Woman drew my blood and sent me to the waiting room.

Why do I have to sit out here? Can't I go home now? I'm tired. It's like two thirty in the morning. I need my beauty sleep. But not as much as you. Just sayin'. Your looks match your personality.

Annoying Woman returned a little later. "You're pregnant."

"No, I'm not." *Flippant giggle.*

"Yes, you are."

"I can't be. I just had my period last week."

"Well, sometimes we still spot when we're pregnant."

"I didn't spot. I had a full-on period." *I think I know what a period looks like. And I think I know what being pregnant feels like.*

"I'm sending you for an ultrasound." She escorted me to another room. Ultrasound Guy came in right away.

I gotta say, the promptness I'm receiving is borderline impressive. He put the jelly stuff on my lower belly, silently checked my uterus, and then walked out of the room. *How rude.*

Doctor walked in.

"Who's your ob-gyn?"

"Dr. Alexander."

"We'll have to call Dr. Alexander and prep you for emergency surgery."

"Pardon me? You're kidding, right?"

"I'm not kidding at all. You have an ectopic pregnancy."

"What does that mean?"

"Your baby is in your fallopian tube and the tube ruptured. This is very serious."

"Oh."

I kid you not, within minutes I was being wheeled down a hallway and was instructed to say goodbye to my husband. *What?! Why would they tell me that? That's a horrible thing to say!*

"So I might *DIE*?"

"There is a definite possibility of death, so you should say goodbye."

I handed Michael my engagement and wedding rings and said, "Give my rings to Greyson for his future wife and tell him I love him, that I'm so proud to be his mom, that he is capable of anything, that I'll watch over him, and to please be a good man." (Justifiable run-on sentence.) Then we exchanged tear-filled declarations of love. And that was that. They gave me about thirty seconds to say goodbye. *Beyond rude.*

As I was being wheeled into the operating room, a very, very attractive Indian man walked alongside me and introduced himself. *Did I die and go to heaven?* He said he was going to be my anesthesiologist. *Thank you, Jesus.* I told him he looked too young to be an anesthesiologist. Seriously, he looked about twenty-five. And beautiful. He responded that this was his very first surgery and gave me a little smile and a wink. Strangely enough, his joke calmed me down, and I happily drifted off into la-la land. *It was a joke, right?*

Well, I lived. If I didn't, you'd be reading a much better

book right now. Apparently, I was two months pregnant. They had to remove my fallopian tube and the baby, but I lived. I was so sad. I'd lost an actual baby. I didn't feel like I'd lost a baby because I'd only known I was pregnant for like twenty minutes, but I did, in fact, lose a baby. I wondered if the baby was a boy or a girl. I wondered what we would've named him or her. I wondered what he or she would've looked like. Would she have been a cheerleader like me or good at every sport like Michael? Would he have been quiet and congenial like Michael or socially awkward but later charming and hilarious like me? I'd never know—until I die too. Then I'll see my son or daughter and immediately know that's him or her. We'll have a lot of catching up to do. Until then my sweet baby.

VIOLET

2008–2009

*B*y April 2008, two months had passed since the miscarriage, and guess what . . . I was pregnant. Again! Baby in uterus. No whooshing of blood. No period or spotting—not that I'd know the difference. Ugh.

We found out it was a girl. We were superexcited. And by we, I mean Michael and me, because as you can imagine, Greyson had the enthusiasm of a sack of potatoes. I was especially delighted because autism was a little less likely in girls. My parents only had two grandchildren at the time; both were boys, and both were autistic. I was hoping a girl would break this trend. *Pretty please, Lord. Pretty please with a cherry on top!*

I'd prayed every night of my life, but after I found out I was pregnant, I begged more than I prayed. *Please Lord, bless me with a girl who is sweet. Please Lord, let her be mentally and physically healthy. Please Lord, let her be happy. Please. Pleeeeeeeease!!!*

With this pregnancy, I was careful like I was with Greyson, but I wasn't over-the-top-fruits-and-vegetables-only-all-natural-everything-no-soda-no-coffee-no-caffeine-no-chocolate-no-fun careful. With Greyson, I was 100 percent committed to a perfect diet. With this pregnancy, I craved plain cheese pizza—which was totally weird because I usually liked toppings. Lots of toppings. Like supercombo, meat-lover toppings. Extra olives. Imagine a dump truck backing up to a pizza and unloading a mountain of toppings. That's how I liked my pizza. But not now. Now I was like, "Cheese only, please." Totally weird. I would also drink a solitary Coke with my pizza. But *only* when I had pizza—which was maybe twice a week. I also craved McDonald's french fries. So, basically, I ate like a three-year-old. This time around, I also allowed myself to have chocolate. I figured I'd been so careful with Greyson, and yet, he was diagnosed with autism, among other things, so what's the diff? I didn't get too crazy. I still cut out alcohol (obviously), coffee, lunch meat, anything containing raw eggs, most preservatives, and most junk food. And I did make a conscious effort to balance my toddler-like cravings with lots of fruits and vegetables.

Like with Greyson, I had every intention of having a natural childbirth, even though the pain was excruciating. So when we got to the hospital on the big day and the nurse asked me if I wanted an epidural, I said I wasn't planning on it. But she asked me if I'd like to meet the anesthesiologist and ask him some questions, so I said, "Sure, why not?"

In walked the dreamy Indian anesthesiologist—the same one who'd put me under for my surgery. *Does my hair look okay? I hope I'm not too sweaty from my contractions.* I told him I remembered him from my surgery, and I thanked him for helping save my life. Then I told him he could stick his needle in me anytime. Nah, . . . just kidding. I didn't say that. I just thought it. There was something about that anesthesiologist I liked, I mean besides his gorgeous face. He made me feel comfortable. So I said yes. *I'll take one epidural, please!*

Weeeee! Epidurals are SO much better than actual real childbirth. No comparison. Not even close. I just sat there, comfortably playing cards with Michael until my doctor eventually told me to push, and I was like, "No problem, dude." Then out popped Violet. Violet Novalee. We still loved the name Novalee after seeing the movie *Where the Heart Is.* The nurse told me Violet looked Chinese, and I don't know if that was a compliment or not because the nurse was Chinese. Either way, Chinese babies are totally adorable, so I took it as a compliment, albeit an inappropriate compliment. In all honesty, Violet didn't come out as beautiful as Greyson. Greyson was the most beautiful baby I'd ever seen. Violet just looked like a baby—a Chinese baby, apparently.

But the best part was that Violet cried when she was born. And when she cried, to me it was like angels singing because Greyson never cried when he was born, which was the first sign, in my opinion, that there was something wrong. It took her a minute, but I sat there begging, "Please cry, please cry, please cry, please cry, please cry," and when she finally did, I was like, "Yes!" Probably not the reaction the doctor was expecting.

The doctor seemed to take forever stitching me up. It was like he was weaving a fucking basket. I was thinking, *What did you do to me?* With Greyson, I didn't have a single stitch! I figured that I shouldn't need stitches with my second baby if I didn't with my first—and Greyson was a bigger baby. And, if I *did* need stitches, then I thought I should only need one, maybe two. Damn stupid doctor cut me almost all the way to my butthole—like dangerously close to my butthole. Just so the bastard could charge my insurance company for an extensive episiotomy. *Can't get as much money without a twenty-five-stitch episiotomy, can you dickhead?* He probably got paid per stitch. He didn't even try *not* to slice me. He just sliced me like a piece of meat. *I bet if I were your wife, I wouldn't need all these stitches, would I?* Needless to say, I was back to hating doctors—except that cute anesthesiologist, of course.

More great news about Violet was that she nursed. It took an hour with a lactation specialist, but she did it! This was another good sign that Violet would be okay.

The next item on my checklist that loosely predicted whether my newborn was autistic or not was her sleep habits. Greyson woke up every hour for eighteen months and still had difficulty sleeping. I firmly believe there's a definite link between mental illness and sleep disorders. So imagine my excitement when, at four months old, Violet was sleeping through the night. That's the typical age for breastfed babies to sleep through the night.

Finally, the most crucial item on my checklist: the smile. Every day I was like, *Smile, smile, smile, smile, smile, smile, smile, smile, smile, smile, smile, SMILE. Smile, dammit!* Violet wasn't an early smiler. She may have even been a late smiler. Maybe my smiling-criteria was too stringent. I didn't want to accidentally count a gassy smile for a smile-smile. I didn't want to set myself up for disappointment. I didn't count it until it was absolutely, positively a smile, which happened about the same time she slept through the night. Greyson was a teenager by this time, and he could still only muster an awkward, forced smile.

Woo-hoo! When Violet was four months old, I unofficially, officially proclaimed that she was not autistic according to Claire's not-at-all-crazy, made-up checklist.

I relished my three-month-long maternity leave from teaching and cuddled and kissed Violet relentlessly. I had to go back to work in mid-April, but I was able to handle it because my amazing mother came from California to live with us and care for Violet until my last day of school in early June. *I can do this. I can go back to work without completely falling apart knowing that in less than two months, I'll have the whole summer to spend with Violet.* Plus, my mom adored her first and only granddaughter and loved having this special time with her.

Greyson also, surprisingly, took a liking to Violet. He would occasionally spend time with her and look at her lovingly-ish. When he held her, he'd generate as close to a happy look as he was able to. Violet took a liking to Greyson too. She seemed happy and content when he was around. It filled my heart to see my favorite boy hold my sweet girl. When Greyson would sit on the floor and play with her, I beamed with pride. *I can't wait for Violet to witness the amazing things her big brother will accomplish in the future,* I thought, *like curing cancer, curing AIDS, discovering a planet.* Although, I knew Greyson's future accomplishments would most likely be those reached alone in a lab versus those that required a vivacious personality or the accompaniment of others. I was pretty sure a profession as a talk-show host was off the table —or anything in customer service or human resources or sales or public relations, basically anything involving humans. Still, I envisioned myself telling Violet, "See what happens when you work hard in school," as I'd revel in the fact that I'd raised an astounding, complex man who made a vast imprint on the ground we call life. I believed with every fiber of my being that God doesn't give a brain like Greyson's to just anyone. That would be a catastrophic waste. God doesn't make mistakes. God has something very special, very monumental planned for Greyson. Plus, I just knew Greyson would ultimately grow out of this autism, sensory processing disorder, and oppositional defiant disorder nonsense. He'd already improved so much. He hadn't physically attacked me in years. And he wore jeans that I didn't even have to cut the tags out of anymore. When I asked Greyson to be Violet's godfather, he thought that was pretty cool . . . I think.

By this time, the gifted program at school kept Greyson busy with loads of homework—like five hours a night. He was taking college-level courses, so I guess that came with the territory. Since Greyson was in a *highly* gifted program in high school versus just a plain ole *gifted* program in middle school, he was finally surrounded by kids who were almost as smart as him. Greyson was finally having conversations with other kids without being completely annoyed by their supposed ignorance. That opened a door for Greyson. He made a friend. Two actually. One was a closeted gay boy from Texas who was living with his born-again Christian parents. Lord bless that boy when he comes out to them. His other new friend was a boy from India whose parents insisted he become a surgeon, but he secretly wanted to be a treasure hunter.

"Like a pirate? Arrrrgh!" I joked.

He looked at me unamused and said, "Yes, kind of like a pirate."

Then I realized he wasn't kidding.

Both were very nice boys, and I prayed their charm would rub off on Greyson. Needless to say, I was way too excited about his friendships and pressured Greyson all the time, "Why don't you invite them over? See if they want to go to the movies. Ask them if they want to work on that project. Do they want to come over for dinner? Do they like filet mignon?" Wait . . . Indians don't eat beef. . . . But maybe Chicago Indians do. What can I do? What can I do? What can I do to make sure you keep your friends? Something . . . anything!

Freshman year, Greyson finally entered the just-make-my-favorite-meal-and-buy-me-video-games stage for his birthday. But we still had a huge Halloween bash, which enjoyed another big turnout. As I walked around the party pretending to make sure kids were good on food and drinks, I watched Greyson interact with the others. As I listened and watched Greyson around his peers, I cringed. He constantly corrected what people said and did strange things like screaming while bashing his head with packing material he'd found in the garage. I could hear that song from *Sesame Street* playing in my head, "One of these things is not like the others. One of these things doesn't belong." *Oh Greyson, how I wish I could help you. How I wish, more than anything, I could magically make you normal.* I'd eventually grown out of my awkwardness—although mine was not accompanied by multiple diagnoses—but hopefully, miraculously, Greyson would too.

On the bright side—the side of me that overflowed with faith in Greyson—he still managed to bring home impressive report cards. Every night as he worked on his homework—which appeared to be written in some sort of code or unrecognizable language—I was like, "Hey Greyson, need some help with that physics thingy?"

"Nope."

Oh, thank God. I'll stick with kindergarten-level instruction.

My kindergarten teaching job was still amazing. I loved it so much, but I found myself counting down the days, hours, and minutes until summer break. It was so difficult to be away from my sweet baby girl, but I was so grateful to have a job with several vacation days built in throughout the year in addition to summers off. Teaching is the perfect job for moms.

This school year I had another wonderful principal. Her name was Diane, and I loved her. She was beautiful, brilliant, and an amazing public speaker. Before every assembly or school event, she would get up in front of hundreds of people and speak with such grace and professionalism that I just sat there in awe. In my eyes, she could do no wrong. I may have had a girl crush on her—her and Kelly Clarkson. I always got a little nervous when I talked to her, even though she was so sweet to me. After I returned from my maternity leave, she called me into her office and said, "Back when I was teaching, once I had children, I always had one hand on the exit door every day at three. I just waited for that bell to ring so I could get home to my kids. I still managed to get everything done even though I left at three." That was her way of saying, "You've always put in long hours for your students, now it's time for you to enjoy your baby." She had faith that I could still do a great job even if I left early. She wanted me to know that she wouldn't be disappointed if I put my family first. That was one of the nicest things anyone had ever done for me.

Diane's children were grown by that time, and she had one daughter away at college majoring in education. When her daughter came home to visit, Diane had her observe me teach a couple times. She also had her attend my end-of-the-year kindergarten show. I was extremely flattered that my principal chose me to be a teacher her daughter observed. Diane also gave me flawless reviews. So did my last principal, Tim. I scored in the excellent range in every single category, every single year. Both Tim and Diane told me they weren't supposed to do that. Apparently, no teacher was excellent at everything—except me. Ha! I received so many excellent reviews from principals and so many letters of appreciation from parents that I made a scrapbook out of them. Only about 10 percent of my parent letters fit in the scrapbook, so I have a box full of them too. "Extra! Extra! Read all about it! Shitty Student Becomes Beloved Teacher!"

PRETEND PEOPLE AND PLACES

2010

*I*n February 2010, I found out I was pregnant ... again.

Michael and I both wanted another girl so badly, but this baby was a boy. I'm ashamed to say that I cried when the ultrasound technician told me. We were just so scared to have another boy because Violet was so easy, and Greyson was so ... Greyson.

After a few years filled with bright flickers of hope—gifted programs, college-level courses, a couple friends (kinda), and no physical episodes—Greyson's behavior became extremely concerning. He'd officially entered the stage where the thought of spending time with Michael or me caused him great dismay. I continued to try and spend time with him by taking him out to lunch, a movie, anything. My attention had primarily shifted to Violet, but I made a conscious effort to let Greyson know that even though I was busy with his sister, I was never too busy to spend time with him. I reminded Greyson that he and I have a special, unbreakable bond that I would never share with anyone else. He was my first baby, and it was just the two of us for so long and those years were precious to me. I'd secretly tell Greyson that he'd always be my favorite because when your children are fourteen years apart, you know by the time the baby could understand what that meant, the older one would be too mature to repeat it. I just wanted Greyson to know that I loved him with all my heart, but he always seemed to turn a deaf ear.

Despite my constant efforts, Greyson's teenagerness became increasingly disturbing and, for lack of a better word, ick. When you take autism, oppositional defiant disorder, and sensory processing disorder and mix 'em all up with raging teenage hormones, then presto chango, you've got one helluva pain in the ass. You think a normal teenager sucks? Greyson was like suckiness on crack. Every moment I spent with him, I had to walk on eggshells just trying not to piss him off. Greyson upgraded his beat-the-crap-out-of-people episodes with his new and improved Scary as Fuck (SAF) episodes, which became increasingly volatile. A pissed-off Greyson was a terrifying Greyson. If I asked him to do something strenuous, like put his shoes away for instance, it would turn into an hour of him disavowing his responsibility in said action. If I didn't cave or express agreement, Greyson got heated. That's when things got scary as fuck.

As Greyson's rage elevated, his clammy face would turn red and his eyes would roll back in his head, showing mostly only white. His body would shake, and his menacing voice would quiver and methodically speak at me. When I would attempt to respond, his body shook harder and the sides of his face dripped with sweat as he raised his voice over mine. If I tried again, he would scream at me with his entire body, which, at that point, would be shaking violently, causing the veins in his strained neck to pulsate.

Not only did he make it clear that my words would never

be heard, but he also followed me to continue his rant if I ignored him or walked away. Similar to when Greyson was younger, he had a difficult time snapping out of this state, which caused his episodes to last at least forty-five minutes, but sometimes, they went on for hours. I had to take my tippy-toeing-around-Greyson skills to the next level. I'd agree with all his ridiculous standpoints. I'd never express an opinion in any way, shape, or form. I'd never ask him to do anything that required effort. When he'd ask me to do something, I would promptly deliver. That was the only way to keep his SAF episodes to a minimum. When I followed that formula, he had maybe one or two SAF episodes a month. When Greyson did have an SAF episode, Michael and I became frightened. Not just a little frightened, though—we were afraid for our lives. And, more importantly, for Violet's life. I often tried to convince myself that Greyson would never hurt Violet. He seemingly loved her, but I never felt sure inside. Not sure enough to believe that he wouldn't hurt her. When we had Violet's crib in our room, we would just lock our bedroom door at night. But after I moved Violet to her own bedroom, I began questioning if Greyson was capable of hurting her. On days when Greyson had an SAF episode, I'd dragged the mattress from the guest bedroom into Violet's bedroom and sleep next to her with the door locked.

The gifted program that Greyson was enrolled in was housed in a wing of a traditional high school with thousands of students, so he still had access to football games and dances. Just as he began showing an interest in social events, his behavior became increasingly peculiar. Greyson would do things like tell me he wanted to go to a high school football game, but then he'd give me the wrong location. After I'd drive across town, he'd insist that the location must've changed because he could never be wrong.

Another time, he wanted to go to a school dance. Alone. I was just happy he wanted to do something social, but when I pulled up to drop him off, everyone was formally dressed, and Greyson was wearing a T-shirt and jeans. When I mentioned that he was underdressed, he just rolled his eyes and hopped out of the car. Then he tried to go inside, but he couldn't because he was supposed to purchase tickets ahead of time. He insisted the school never announced that tickets had to be purchased in advance or that the dance was formal, even though eight hundred other kids managed to show up in dresses and ties with tickets in hand. And back then, there were no smartphones or fancy school websites for me to confirm his last-minute plans.

Repeatedly, Greyson would tell me that a "friend" had invited him over, so I'd drive him to their house just to find out no one was there. "Why did he ask me to come over if he's not home?" he'd say. He'd also constantly give me incorrect directions to various places and insist he was misinformed. Greyson never took ownership for any errors or mistakes he made. If I ever asked for a phone number to verify directions or confirm our arrival beforehand, he'd refuse. "Don't be ridiculous, Mom," he'd say with extreme irritation. I knew arguing would lead to an SAF episode, so I continued to drive him to empty homes and empty football fields so I could sleep in my own bed at night instead of on Violet's floor.

Then there were the times when he'd demand at ten o'clock on a school night, "Take me to Walgreens. I need something for a project." I didn't dare bring up the fact that we'd passed two Walgreens five hours earlier when we ran to Target, which, by the way, also had the supplies he needed. Greyson liked to wait until the night before to begin his school projects. His severe procrastination, lack of common sense, and poor sleep habits always seemed to affect me. But if I ever mentioned any of this to him, it would turn into an unwinnable hour-long argument and an SAF episode. So I'd get my pregnant ass out of bed and drive to Walgreens in my pajamas.

Up until this point, Greyson had always been very responsible in specific areas. He'd always gotten straight As, always kept a spotless room, was superorganized, and was always on time. But all of a sudden, he was constantly missing the bus because he'd overslept. When this occurred, he'd matter-of-factly say, "Aren't you going to drive me to school?" in a tone that implied it was my duty—as if I didn't have a job to get to or anything to do in the morning with a toddler.

Greyson also missed the bus after school occasionally. When he did this, he'd use the phone in the school office to call me. "You have to come get me."

Well, hello to you too. "At school?"

"Yes. Right now."

"How do you miss the bus when you're already at school and just have to walk from your classroom to your locker to the bus?"

Click.

One particular time, I hustled from work to Greyson's school and pulled up to the main entrance—exactly where I'd always pulled up when he missed the bus—but there was no Greyson. So I sat there and sat there for fifteen minutes. Still, no Greyson. At that point, I parked my car, went into the school, and searched for him for twenty minutes. No Greyson. So I went back to my car and sat there waiting for him, as if I had absolutely nothing else to do with my time and just loved hanging out in my car doing nothing. *Oy vey.* After twenty minutes, I got out of the car and started walking around the campus. Finally, I found Greyson lying on the ground in some tall grass about a hundred feet away from where I normally picked him up.

"What are you doing? I've been here for an hour looking for you. Did you even bother to lift your head six inches to see if my car was sitting there in that empty parking lot?"

"Nope."

As much as I enjoyed driving to pretend places to see pretend people and spending pointless hours in my car, I wanted Greyson to learn how to drive so my desire to murder him would lessen. After Greyson completed driving school and got his permit, I let him drive one morning after he'd missed the bus yet again.

"Greyson, you just backed out of the garage without looking first."

"I'm just backing up, I don't need to look."

"Greyson, you just rolled through a stop sign."

"No one stops at stop signs."

"When a light turns green, you should look both ways before going, just in case someone runs a red light— especially when you're the first car in line."

"The light was green. Green means go."

After fifteen minutes of pure horror that I'm pretty sure shaved years off my life, Greyson pulled into the parking lot and hit a curb. Of course, that wasn't his fault, either, because why was that curb there anyway? Greyson was always right and knew everything about everything. He was an expert driver and street designer, and the rules of the road were just suggestions.

Yes, there was so much fun being had at that time. But wait, there's more!

Greyson also started to become very uncharacteristically messy and careless. Greyson had never been messy or careless a day in his life. His room had been spotless and organized since birth. He was probably the only child in existence who'd never lost a single puzzle or game piece, even though he owned hundreds of puzzles and games. But all of a sudden, Greyson was doing things like ruining his bathroom countertop. One time, while my parents were visiting, Greyson was working on a project that required the use of Gorilla Glue. I asked my dad if he knew what had happened when I discovered large clear globs scattered all over the countertop in Greyson's bathroom. My dad told me he'd noticed Greyson working on a project using Gorilla Glue, so he said, "Greyson, you have to put something under your project to protect the counter." When my dad checked on Greyson later, he noticed that he'd put a single piece of toilet paper under his large project. So my dad handed Greyson some newspaper and reminded him that he had to protect the countertop. Later that evening, my dad saw Greyson finishing up his project with the newspaper sitting on the floor. That never would've happened with ten-year-old Greyson or even three-year-old Greyson.

In case you're wondering, Gorilla Glue does not come off. I even called the company. No luck.

Now as unexpected as all these new characteristics were, I was not at all prepared for what came next: Greyson's grades started to drop—dramatically. He went from earning straight As with ease his entire life to earning below-average grades. By the end of his sophomore year of high school, Greyson no longer qualified for the gifted program, so he couldn't take college-level classes. This was the unforeseen straw that broke the camel's back. I lied and told Greyson it was time for his annual school physical then called the doctor and told her I wanted Greyson tested for drugs.

The test came back negative. So what exactly was causing Greyson to become careless, messy, late, lazy, delusional, and even more defiant and scarier than usual? Nothing made sense. That was the year I started questioning what was in store for Greyson. I started praying every night that Greyson would have the successful life I'd envisioned for so long. I also began praying for something I never thought imaginable. I prayed every night that my unborn son would be nothing like Greyson. Nothing. I hoped he'd be 180 degrees different than Greyson. *Lord, please let this baby be the exact opposite of Greyson. Greyson has never been happy, and I want this baby to be happy. Greyson has never had friends; I want this baby to be surrounded by friends. Greyson is so defiant and difficult; I want this baby to be loving and sweet. Greyson has never been liked; I want everyone to like this baby.* It broke my heart to ask God for such things.

ROCKWELL

2010

*I*n October 2010, a couple of months after Greyson turned sixteen, I went into labor. Throughout this pregnancy, I'd craved cheeseburgers. Cheeseburgers, cheeseburgers, cheeseburgers. I may or may not have eaten four or five a week. It's funny how I craved totally different foods with all three pregnancies. Fortunately, I still loved fruits and vegetables, so I managed to balance my diet. When it comes to food, I live by the 80/20 rule: 80 percent healthy, 20 percent fun. During this pregnancy, my diet was 80 percent healthy, 20 percent cheeseburgers.

We went to the hospital around eleven o'clock at night. I didn't realize at the time what a disadvantage it was to go into labor at bedtime. I was put in a hospital room and my assigned nurse, who wasn't very friendly, asked if I wanted an epidural. I didn't rule it out because it was so blissful when I'd given birth to Violet, so I told her I wasn't sure.

She sent in the anesthesiologist, but he wasn't dreamy like my last anesthesiologist. I told him I needed time to decide.

The nurse came back in and said I had until one o'clock in the morning to decide because the anesthesiologist was leaving for the night. She said getting an epidural would speed up the delivery.

"I'm not sure." I told her.

"You have until one o'clock," she snapped.

I don't like you.

I didn't like Michael at the moment either. While staring at the clock, he kept asking me if I'd made a decision yet. Like my decision affected him. *Stop pressuring me. You're supposed to be rubbing my back, feeding me ice chips, and lying to my face telling me how beautiful I look.*

I kept thinking about how Greyson's birth was so torturous and Violet's birth was so heavenly. I thought about how epidurals have been around forever and millions of women manage to survive them. I thought about how I'd never personally met a woman from my generation who didn't get an epidural during childbirth. I mean, I know they're out there, but I've never actually known one. Between my friends, my teacher friends, and my husband's friends, I'd never once come across someone who said, "Yeah, I decided against an epidural." In fact, whenever it came up in conversation that I'd had Greyson naturally, people looked at me like I was insane and seemed confused by my stupidity. I tried explaining to myself that having a hot anesthesiologist was not actually the reason why my last epidural was so great.

My annoying nurse continued to pop in every twenty minutes to ask if I'd made a decision yet—like she made a commission for every epidural sold. Or maybe there was an epidural contest of some sort, like a traveling epidural trophy. Perhaps a coveted Mirrorball balanced on a giant gold needle. I couldn't understand why it was so damn important to her that I got an epidural.

Eventually, I caved and said yes—anything just to shut her (and Michael) up. I just wanted everyone to shut up and leave me alone. I wanted to blissfully wait for my baby to arrive like I'd done with Violet. Maybe take in a movie and occasionally glance at the screen that showed I was having a contraction and be like, *Take that contraction. Can't even feel you beotch!*

Dr. UnMcDreamy returned and proceeded to give me the epidural. As with my past anesthesiologist, I told him that I was very sensitive to medicine and to give me the lowest dosage. Then, *POOF*, he was gone. I got the feeling he was annoyed by my indecisiveness. Perhaps he could've left work early had I not taken so long to decide.

Finally, the nurse left me alone, and Michael went to sleep. All was good, all was quiet . . . for about fifteen minutes.

I pressed that little red button in my room—you know, the button they tell you to press if you need anything. The nurse walked in like *I* was the one bothering *her*. Clearly, she was in the lead for the epidural trophy and no longer wanted to be bothered. "I think there's something wrong with my epidural. My face feels strange."

She glanced at the machine I was hooked up to.

"All looks good. You're fine. You should get some sleep."

"Some sleep? I thought the epidural was going to speed things up?"

"It will, but for now, you should get some rest. You need some sleep before the baby comes," and out she walked.

Hmm. Okay. Well, sleep was the last thing I was going to get. My face felt really weird, and I didn't feel relaxed like I did with Violet. Something wasn't right. I pressed the red button again. "I think my dosage needs to be turned down, I really don't feel right."

"The anesthesiologist left and the doctor is sleeping. I'm sure you're fine. Get some rest."

Twenty minutes later, I pressed the red button.

"*Yeeees?*" the nurse griped, clearly irritated by my button pressing.

By this point, I was in tears. "I'm sure something is wrong! I need someone to help me! This is not how an epidural is supposed to feel!"

"Do you know your leg is hanging off the table?" she asked.

"No, I didn't know. Again, I need someone to help me. Please get my doctor."

"Your doctor is asleep."

"This isn't how my epidural felt with my daughter."

"Did you give birth at this hospital?"

"No."

"Well, we use a different brand of medicine, and people react differently to different brands. I'm sure that's it. You'll be fine."

Twenty minutes later. Red button.

"Yeeeeeeeeees?"

Now crying hysterically, "I really need a doctor! I know something is wrong!"

"Well, if I get the doctor, and he turns down your dosage, then you're going to feel a lot of pain. You really should leave it the way it is. The anesthesiologist knows what he's doing. You'll be fine."

"But I'm *not* fine! It doesn't feel right!"

"It *is* right. You'll be fine."

Now all you have to do is read what I just wrote over and over again because that's how my night went. I felt like I was trapped in the movie *Misery* and Kathy Bates was my nurse. I cried and screamed hysterically for seven solid hours, pressing that fucking useless red button over and over while being assured I was fine. That bitch told me I was fine so many times that I began to believe her. I started to think I was making a big deal over nothing—that their brand of epidural just didn't "agree" with me like the other brand. Kind of like coffee creamer. For some reason, certain brands of coffee creamer hurt my stomach while others don't. It's *JUST* like that—the same exact fucking thing!

Never in my life had I felt so abandoned, helpless, and insignificant as I did that night. No one was there for me: not my nurse, not my doctor, not the anesthesiologist, and certainly not my husband who slept through it all.

Around eight o'clock in the morning, the doctor sauntered into my room.

Good morning fuckface. Did you have a pleasant slumber? So nice of you to join me.

About forty-five minutes later, my son was born. By then, there were several nurses in the room, and they'd suddenly started acting strangely exhilarated, yelling numbers like they were at the stock exchange.

"Eleven!"

"Ten-nine!"

"Eleven-three!"

Then the doctor joined in, "Ten-five!"

What's happening? Is there some sort of emergency? What's wrong?

The baby cried.

Yes! Yes! Yes! I wasn't sure if I should be happy or freaking out, but, yay, he cried!

The doctor placed my boy on the scale and yelled, "Ten on the nose!" Then they all threw their arms up and cheered.

Weight? They were guessing my baby's weight! Did he just say ten pounds? Who's baby is ten pounds? Certainly not mine. I don't have ten-pound babies. Seven is my number. Eight, tops!

"Here you go, Tank, meet your mama," a nurse said as she handed me a baby that couldn't have possibly just come out of my vagina.

He looks six months old! What the heck? He looks, he looks . . . amazing. Something happened in that moment that I can't quite describe. I had this feeling that I'd just given birth to my best friend. Like I wanted to take him out for a beer and shoot the shit. Like he was my guy, my buddy. My fear of autism instantly melted away, and I just knew: this was my guy, my little dude.

His Apgar score was a ten—a perfect baby. One nurse told me she'd never seen a baby get a ten, "I've seen some nines, but never a ten. Didn't think they gave tens."

I literally gave birth to a ten. Me!

Over the next few hours, every nurse that came to check on him referred to him as Tank. I felt so proud—like Wonder Woman. *Yeah, I gave birth to that.*

"What are you going to name him?" asked a nurse.

"Rockwell. Rockwell Remington."

"Rockwell. I can't think of a better name for Tank. Good job." Then she gave me a wink.

Why couldn't you have been my nurse last night?

For the sole purpose of proving that the doctor who delivered Violet gave me an episiotomy just so he could get more money for my delivery, I'd like to mention that with ten-pound Rockwell, I did not have one single stitch. With Greyson, I did not have one single stitch. Apparently, my vagina is part rubber band. However, with my middle child— my smallest baby with no delivery complications—I had twenty-five stitches.

I eventually regained feeling in my legs although it took an abnormally long time. I still felt off, but it was camouflaged by my extreme feeling of joy that I'd given birth to the coolest kid ever born. He was so cute too. No, *cute* is the wrong word. He looked like a stud—like he should be leaving the hospital wrapped in a biker jacket and sunglasses instead of a pale blue receiving blanket and a beanie. *He don't*

*need no stinkin' beanie. He wants to feel the wind blow through his
hair.*

Since I'd earned Wonder Woman status in the hospital, I
didn't think much of it when I brushed my teeth and couldn't
hold or swish the water in my mouth. Or that when I drank
water, it dribbled out of my mouth. I didn't have much time
to think about it anyway since I left the hospital about seven
hours after Rockwell was born. And after such a traumatic
night, I was ready to ditch that dump.

Within a day, I started noticing the difficulties I was
having with eating and drinking. I called my doctor's office
and spoke to a nurse and told her my symptoms. The nurse
told me to go to the emergency room.

"What? The emergency room?" I was not expecting that
response. "Ask the doctor, please."

One minute later.

"He said you need to go to the emergency room
immediately!"

"Immediately?" *Immediately is not really a good time for me.
You see, I actually just got home from the hospital.*

"You have to go right now. Not tomorrow. Now!"

"Why?"

"These are signs that you've had a stroke."

"A *WHAT*!?"

So off I went to the emergency room, leaving my one-
day-old breastfed baby behind. The good news was that
when I arrived, there were a thousand people there. That was
good news because when I told them my symptoms, they
took me into a room instantly. I'm not gonna lie—there's
something gratifying about dodging a five-hour wait.

When I walked into the room, the doctor took one look
at me and said, "You've got Bell's palsy."

"Bell's palsy?"

"The left side of your face is paralyzed."

That's when I started ugly-crying, even though I knew nothing about Bell's palsy.

"Don't worry. It's highly likely that you'll regain feeling in your face within three months."

Don't worry?! Highly likely?! Three months?! "It was my epidural. I knew something was wrong! I told the nurse I could feel it in my face, but she wouldn't listen!"

"There's no medical evidence that links epidurals to Bell's palsy."

No medical evidence?! No medical evidence, my ass. I'm *medical evidence.* It was so blatantly obvious that my epidural caused it. Have I mentioned that I loathe doctors? And nurses. And anesthesiologists.

I cried, and drooled, all the way home.

The next day my mom showed up at my door. That's when the real fugly crying began. I'd never been so happy to see someone in my life. She came to cheer me up and help me with Violet and Rockwell. I sure needed my mom right then.

My maternity leave was whizzing by, and my face was still paralyzed. Michael and I sat down to discuss what I should do. Together, we decided that I should take the remainder of the school year off. We were considering it even before a paralyzed face was a variable, but having Bell's palsy sealed the deal. Rockwell was born in October, so I worked less than two months that school year. I felt such relief and happiness when we made the decision that I would stay home. I had almost an entire year to just enjoy Violet and Rockwell. Despite the Bell's palsy, that was the best year of my life—except where Greyson was concerned.

At this point, Greyson was sixteen years old and a junior at a traditional high school. After he'd been kicked out of the gifted program, he had to switch to a high school closer to home. At his new school, his grade point average plummeted, even though he considered the classes there "laughable." He wasn't doing any classwork or homework, but he still aced every test, so he managed to maintain a C average. After nearly a decade of straight As, this was a hard pill for me to swallow—especially knowing he was capable of acing college-level courses.

During this time, Greyson did take up a hobby: drumming. When he started showing a little interest in the drums, of course my parents bought him a beautiful drum set when they heard the news. Like me, they got really excited when Greyson made a couple friends or showed interest in . . . well, anything, really. Nothing excited Greyson because he believed everything was beneath him. Greyson became so good at drumming so fast that he joined the school band and was soon named lead drummer, even though he'd only been playing a few months.

Normally, I would've embraced the opportunity to drive Greyson to school functions where he held the title of lead drummer, and I was beyond thrilled that he was actually involved in something. However, when I drove Greyson anywhere, he just sat in silence when I asked about his day. He also continued to give me incorrect information and wrong locations.

"Pick me up at five," he'd say.

I'd arrive promptly at five.

"What are you doing here? I said to pick me up at seven."

Door slams in my face.

Three days later.

"Mom, the game is at Lincoln High School."

"Are you sure?"

Loud sigh, then silence.

Arrived at wrong location—again.

Greyson missed game—again.

Greyson also continued to oversleep, miss the bus, and lose things. "Greyson, I was contacted by the school saying you lost all your textbooks."

"Yep."

"Those books cost hundreds of dollars."

"I don't need them."

"I still have to replace them. They're property of the school."

"If you must."

Greyson continued to become even more disorganized, messy, careless, and lazy. This was particularly annoying because we'd decided to sell our home during the housing market crash.

"Greyson, we got a call about the house and have a showing in an hour. Please empty your trash and clean your bathroom—especially your toilet!"

After Michael and I had cleaned frantically for forty minutes, we noticed that Greyson's bathroom door was shut, and we hadn't heard a peep from him.

"Greyson! What are you doing? Our showing is in twenty minutes!"

"I'm pooping."

"Have you cleaned your bathroom yet?"

"No. I told you. I'm pooping."

"You've been pooping for forty minutes?"

"Yep."

"They'll be here in twenty minutes, Greyson. We really need your help. Please clean your bathroom—especially your toilet! Please!"

Silence.

Michael and I ran around like chickens with our heads

cut off for twenty more minutes. "Greyson! Time to go. We have to leave right now. They just pulled up!"

Greyson tootles downstairs like he's got nowhere to be.

"Let's go! They're here!"

We headed to the park next to our house so Violet could play and Rockwell could swing during the one-hour scheduled showing. When we arrived back home, I was proud of how beautiful our home looked considering that we'd only had an hour to prepare with two little kids. When I made my way upstairs, I peeked into Greyson's bathroom. Not only did he not clean it at all, but he left his giant poop in the toilet. He didn't even bother to flush!

"You have got to be kidding me, Greyson! The toilet is full of poo, and it smells repulsive in here! How embarrassing! All I asked was that you clean your bathroom! Michael and I cleaned the entire rest of the house!"

"A little poo in the toilet won't make a difference."

"*A LITTLE POO* won't make a difference?! *A LITTLE POO* won't make a difference?!" I screamed.

Michael ran upstairs and saw the poo-filled toilet, overflowing garbage can, toothpaste-covered sink, and water-spotted mirror. Michael was typically careful about avoiding SAF episodes, but this time, he couldn't hold back from giving Greyson a piece of his mind.

Greyson talked over Michael as if he weren't even speaking.

"I. HAD. TO. POO. I. HAD. TO. POO." Greyson screamed over and over, louder and louder, as his face turned beet red. His voice trembled. His body shook. His eyes rolled back. His stare looked menacing. Then he screamed, "Fuck you!," and I thought we were going to die from toothbrush-induced stab wounds.

Greyson's SAF episode lasted about an hour. Even though we removed ourselves from the bathroom, we continued to hear him occasionally scream that he'd had to poo. I made sure not to leave Violet or Rockwell unattended the rest of the day. Then, like I had when Violet was a baby, I dragged the spare mattress—and now Rockwell too—into her room where I locked the door and slept on the floor with the kids that night. I was so tired of feeling scared in my own home. Tired of worrying about Violet and Rockwell's safety. That was the reason why we'd decided to sell our home during the worst housing market crash in history. We had to move to be more separated from Greyson. We weren't even sure what that looked like yet, but the older Greyson got, the more fearful Michael and I became of him. That was the year I completely stopped being excited about Greyson's future and started being frightened by it.

THE PLEASURE IS ALL MINE, CONNIE

2011

*I*t took about four months, but by February 2011 my face was no longer paralyzed. I continued to feel residual effects (that have progressively worsened to this day), but I was thrilled that I could eat and drink again without drooling.

The silver lining of having Bell's palsy was that I got to be at home with Violet and Rockwell, which I enjoyed more than anything in the world. Even though we were falling into debt without my income, Michael and I agreed that I should take another year off. I knew my babies would only be little once, and I wanted to enjoy those critical years. Since I had the best job in the world, an additional year of maternity leave was approved. That was without pay, of course, but my job was guaranteed for the following school year. Nothing has ever made me happier than being with my babies every day. They were both so sweet, but so different.

Violet was so loving, expressive, sweet, and cuddly. She had a stuffed dog named Puppy that she slept with and carried around the house. Puppy was not allowed outside because he was much too valuable. Mommy spent hours looking for a backup Puppy, but he was extinct. Violet sucked her thumb when she cuddled Puppy, and Puppy was cuddled so much that he looked like a dishrag. Violet loved stuffed animals and cars; she showed no interest in dolls or princesses. Violet was an easy toddler, but she did have an occasional tantrum. She was also crowned World's Pickiest Eater. Until she was eighteen months old, she would only eat baby food. Anything else I gave her made her gag and give me the how-could-you-do-this-to-me-Mommy face. Then, at eighteen months old, she really broadened her horizons by eating slices of cheese, cubed cheese, string cheese, shredded cheese, cheese pizza, grilled cheese, and macaroni and cheese. Violet was also very smart—not Greyson smart, just a normal level of smart. She knew all her letters shortly after she turned two and was excellent at jigsaw puzzles. When she was thinking, she'd stick out her tongue, like a little Michael Jordan.

Then there was my Rockwell. He and Violet were twenty-one months apart. Rockwell was the easiest baby in the history of the universe. He was so happy, so loving, and so hilarious. He was a little comedian. Rockwell knew he was silly, and he cracked himself up. He was always smiling and always in a good mood. And he was still a butterball. He remained "off the charts" in height and weight. By age one, he was already wearing size 3 clothes. Unlike Violet, Rockwell completely skipped the baby food stage and went straight for the good stuff. When I attempted to give him baby food, he'd spit it out and grab food from my plate. The kid would devour anything I put in front of him. He was a human vacuum.

Raising two sweet, loving, well-behaved children made me realize just how incredibly difficult it was raising Greyson, who, at this time, was sixteen. Since Greyson was my first, I'd never realized quite the extent of how arduous he was. Greyson woke up every hour at night for eighteen straight months and hardly ever napped; Violet and Rockwell had both slept through the night from the time they were four months old and were excellent nappers. It took Greyson five months and five lactation specialists to learn to nurse; Violet and Rockwell nursed at the hospital when they were only a few hours old. Greyson never smiled; Violet and Rockwell always smiled. Greyson never made eye contact; Violet and Rockwell looked right at me and smiled. (It melted my heart—I never knew what I was missing!) Greyson started hitting me a hundred times a day around five months old; Violet and Rockwell, um, never did that. I can't even imagine them doing that. It seemed so bizarre thinking about how Greyson beat the shit out of me every single day at their age. And, for the record, I didn't do anything differently with Violet and Rockwell than I did with Greyson. I was the same loving, attentive mom. There's not a single thing I would change about how I raised Greyson.

The only thing Greyson had missing in his life was Sperm Donor and his family. Then the strangest thing happened. One day in the spring of 2011, I was walking with Violet and pushing Rockwell in a stroller past a restaurant. As I walked by, a woman ran out of the restaurant yelling my name. I turned around, and standing there was Sperm Donor's sister Mary. Ironically, Mary now lived in Chicago. Apparently, the job that sent her to Chicago on a business trip years earlier had transferred her. Mary seemed so excited to see me. *Why's she so happy to see me?* She was acting so bubbly and nice, like I was her long-lost best friend. That really caught me off guard since Mary had acted like I had the plague the last time I'd seen her ten years earlier when she stood up me and Greyson. I spoke to her for a few minutes, very awkwardly I might add, then made up an excuse to leave. Actually, I can't remember a word I said. I felt so discombobulated and annoyed by her disingenuousness. It made me sick. I couldn't believe Mary lived so close to me. At least the rest of them were still in Oklahoma.

I managed to get away from Mary without saying "Here's my e-mail and phone number. Let's keep in touch." But that didn't stop Sperm Donor's mother, Connie, from e-mailing me for the first time EVER a few days later. *So you can find people when you set your mind to it?* Apparently, she was waiting until Greyson was sixteen to swoop in for her Grandmother of the Year award. I had never met or had a conversation with that woman, but she turned out to be insane. *Shocker.* She's a southern born-again Christian. *Of course she is.* Pretending she doesn't have a grandson for sixteen years is *so* born-again Christian-y.

In Connie's e-mail, she claimed that she'd only recently found out about Greyson but would like to have a relationship with him. *She's such a hoot.* I guess Mary failed to mention to her mom that she physically spent an entire day with Greyson ten years ago. I'm sure the subject just never came up, even though they're very close and see each other all the time. Must've just slipped Mary's mind.

Connie expressed in that first e-mail to me that I was "a grown woman who made the personal choice to be sexually involved outside of marriage and made the irresponsible choice to not use birth control." *Well, that's a fine how do you do. I don't remember asking your opinion. And you forgot to mention that your son was there too—your narcissistic, sociopathic son.*

I actually agreed with her statement, but I was baffled that she felt the authority to lecture me. Connie also stated in that very first e-mail to me, "If you do not forgive others of their sins, your Father will not have mercy on you and forgive you of your sins."

Oh my gosh, I was just thinking the exact *same thing!* She's a born-again Christian *and* a mind reader! I think I get it now. All I have to do is forgive Sperm Donor, and God will have mercy on me, and Greyson will no longer suffer. Geez, why didn't you say that sixteen years ago? And why are you lecturing me after sixteen years without knowing whether or not I'd forgiven Sperm Donor and without knowing whether or not *I believed* I'd made an irresponsible choice.

Obviously, I made an irresponsible choice. Duh.

This woman that I'd never met or spoken to was ripping me apart in an e-mail. It's funny how born-again Christians think they're better than everyone else and don't think the rules of society apply to them.

I decided to e-mail her back.

Dear Connie, Fuck you.

Backspace, backspace, backspace.

Dear Connie, What in hell's bells are you smoking?

Backspace, backspace, backspace.

You can do it. Be nice Claire.

Dear Connie,

As I'm sure you are aware, I ran into Mary recently. Hearing from you and seeing Mary reminded me of all the hurt, sadness, and rejection I felt from you, Mary, Michael Sr., and of course, your son. It sickens me to think back to how I reached out to Michael Sr. and his wife when Greyson was little and how they brushed off my invitation to be a part of their grandson's life. Then, ten years ago, I contacted Mary. Greyson and I spent a day with her in Chicago. We made plans to get together the next day, but she stood us up and never called. A few years later, I tried again. When Mary didn't answer my calls, I left a message saying I would really like to at least stay in touch through Christmas cards. I told her to please call me back and tell me her address. I never heard back. Every year at Christmas and on Greyson's birthday, I hoped that you, your son, Michael Sr., or Mary would reach out to us. Greyson never received so much as a card from any of you.

In your e-mail, you accused me of withholding information about you and your family from Greyson. I can assure you that is not the case. I have made it a point to tell Greyson he can talk to me about anything, and I'd be happy to answer any questions regarding his biological father or family. I told Greyson he has three half siblings (that I'm aware of—I left out the "from three different women" part). I even told Greyson I would be happy to take him to Oklahoma to meet anyone. At one point, I actually encouraged Greyson to have a relationship with his half siblings. I explained that they are innocent in all of this. I showed Greyson pictures of his dad and half sister that I received from Mary ten years ago. I have been extremely honest and open with Greyson his whole life. And I've continuously added all my favorite pictures of Greyson to a photo album for your son if he ever showed any interest in Greyson.

It's bothersome that after almost seventeen years of my dedication and sacrifice, you now want to be a part of Greyson's life. Greyson has been an extremely challenging boy to raise, but I can wholeheartedly say I have given him 110 percent of myself. I've loved Greyson since the day I found out I was pregnant. I have been an extremely involved and loving parent. I've never had much money, but Greyson has never been in need of anything. I rarely went out, never bought much for myself, and never once asked your son for a penny. Still, every Christmas and every birthday, I hoped maybe that would be the year he'd send me a check to buy gifts for his son.

Now, after so much heartache, sacrifice, and hard work, you want to stroll into Greyson's life? Life is way too short for me to spend time with people who don't care about my family. Had you contacted me years ago, things would be much different. I wish Greyson could have known you and his Aunt Mary. But I'm afraid your e-mails are too little, too late.

Claire

That was nice of me, right? Considering the circumstances, I think that was pretty fucking nice. But no . . .

Connie responded and accused me of brainwashing Greyson stating, "It is very, very wrong of you to let Greyson think I don't care about him because that is not at all true."

Did you even read my letter, lady? And, is it just me, or maybe (just maybe) you not contacting me for almost seventeen years sums up how much you actually care.

Connie also stated that ten years ago, "Mary couldn't handle my emotional situation." Wait, I thought you didn't know Greyson existed until recently? And yes, I can totally understand how getting a Christmas card from me once a year would be hard for Mary to handle. And yes, I'm a complete emotional wreck. Just ask any parent whose child I've taught, any principal I've worked for, or any professor I had while maintaining straight As in graduate school. They all gave me beautiful letters, evaluations, and grades because they were afraid that if they didn't, I'd *SNAP*! I'm crazy like that.

Oh, oh, oh, and my favorite part was when Connie accused me of "living under assumed names."

Like she needed Sherlock Holmes to find me. Ugh. Being a teacher, I had to get fingerprinted and all my information was public knowledge since I was a government employee. Elementary, my dear Connie.

Lastly, are you ready for this? Connie stated in her e-mails that she too had a baby out of wedlock (at age sixteen) but then said, "The only difference between you and me is that I chose to stand before Jesus Christ and throw myself at His mercy while accepting responsibility for my actions."

Tell her what she's won, Johnny! Um, woman, I'm pretty sure raising Greyson and never asking for a penny of child support is kinda the definition of taking responsibility for my actions. Maybe she's confusing me with her son.

After our thread of e-mails, I felt defeated and angry. So she did her job, just like any good born-again Christian would.

Until then, I'd never realized the ginormous bullet I dodged when Grandma Connie blew us off. *Now that's what I call divine intervention.* I really want to like born-again Christians. I really, really, really do, but they just keep finding ways to prove how nauseating they are.

I decided not to continue our correspondence because I can't handle stupidity. I think we can safely rule out that Greyson got his brilliance from her.

Connie did, however, teach me something: There's one thing worse than born-again Christians and that's stupid born-again Christians.

Of course, I didn't mention to Connie that Greyson was struggling. I didn't even mention it to my parents. They loved him so much, and I didn't want them to worry. They were already concerned when Greyson left the gifted program, but "teenagers will be teenagers."

BOOGERS AND GRAPES

2011–2012

*I*n the fall of 2011, my mom and dad (aka Greyson's normal grandparents) were in town staying with us for several weeks, like they always did two or three times a year. My parents were amazing at making sure they were very present in my kids' lives. Greyson was typically on his best behavior when they were in town because my parents loved having the job of spoiling him. "That's what grandparents are for," they'd say, but my parents were so much more than that.

We only had two showers in our house—one in the master bathroom and one in Greyson's bathroom. My parents were always concerned that they were a bother (which of course they weren't), so they used Greyson's shower when they were in town. My mom brought to my attention that Greyson still had the same bottle of shampoo that he'd had when they'd visited months before.

"How is that possible? Are you sure?"

"Positive."

I went into his bathroom and checked under the sink where I stored backup bottles for when he ran out of shampoo. "Hmm . . . there's two backup bottles down here. Now that you mention it, I guess I haven't bought him shampoo in a while." I looked at the shampoo bottle in his shower. It was barely used.

Later that night, I nonchalantly gave Greyson a kiss on the top of his head while he watched TV. When I took a whiff of his hair, I almost passed out. Later, I casually asked Greyson if he needed more shampoo.

"Nope. I'm good."

I really didn't want Greyson to have an SAF episode with my parents in town, so I decided to keep an eye on his shampoo to make sure he really wasn't using it. I put a little mark at the shampoo line using a Sharpie on the clear bottle.

Since Greyson had become a slob, he'd begun leaving piles of dirty dishes in his room. I hardly recognized his room anymore because he used to be so clean and organized. Then I started to notice little black, brown, and green goops along the edges of the plates that had piled up in his room. I had to scrub and scrape the plates to get them off. *What in the world is this?*

This continued for a month. I'd scrub, I'd scrape, I'd wonder. The only thing the goops really looked like was boogers, but, surely, that wasn't possible.

I waited until my parents left, then I asked Greyson if he was picking his nose and wiping his boogers on his dirty dishes.

"Maybe."

"Maybe?! And who do you think has to scrub and scrape your dried-up boogers off the plates?"

"Dunno."

"Me, Greyson. Me. I'm the one scrubbing and scraping your dried-up boogers off the plates! So if you could stop doing that, I'd really appreciate it."

Silence.

I know what you're thinking, *Why don't you make him scrub and scrape his own boogers off his own plates?* That is soooo I-don't-have-a-mentally-ill-son of you. Here's the thing, you can't make a six-foot-five-inch autistic teenager with oppositional defiant disorder do anything. I was just thrilled when he didn't scream at me for things like putting too many potatoes on his plate for dinner. I use that as an example because he once literally screamed at me for putting too many potatoes on his plate for dinner. I walked on eggshells around Greyson. When I attempted to talk to him or just ask him about his day, he'd walk away.

"Are you just going to walk away from me every time I talk to you?"

Walked away. Turned around. Pointed at my face. And said, "Exactly."

Greyson also became weirdly forgetful about simple everyday tasks. He'd forget to do effortless things like close the front door when he left, take his keys so he could get back in, turn off the oven or stove after cooking, wear shoes to school. Yes, it could be zero degrees outside, and he'd forget to wear shoes to school. He'd also forgot to do things like get his picture taken on picture day and then again on makeup picture day. He wasn't absent those days; he just forgot to go to the auditorium. The other three-thousand students managed to get there, but not Greyson. He just wondered why no one was in class and everyone was in the auditorium. I prepaid fifty bucks for a yearbook without Greyson's picture in it.

Greyson also became very destructive, which was something he never was in the past. He did things including, but not limited to, dropping my video camera down the stairs, ruining our carpet by putting Play-Doh all over it, and breaking our lawn mower because according to him, it's "not a big deal" to mow over rocks or run into trees. When he took his bike out of the garage, he repeatedly, haphazardly allowed his handlebars to drag alongside my car, causing at least fifty deep scratches across the entire length of my car.

After I brought this to his attention for the third time, he bought some five-dollar scratch remover. I told him that he absolutely could not use a five-dollar scratch remover on my car. Then, later that day, he went into the garage and used it all over the side of my car, completely removing the paint. It looked like he'd scrubbed my car with an S.O.S pad. Oddly enough, he refused to admit he was the one who'd scrubbed my car with scratch remover, even after I found the tube with the cap off and the product oozing out—like someone else broke into our garage and tried to buff the scratches on my car. *It must've been the Scratch-Removing Fairy. Or better yet, maybe Violet and Rockwell did it. Two toddlers scrubbing my car with scratch remover makes much more sense.* He argued with me over things like that until I would give up and said something like, "Okay Greyson, I believe you. Someone else must've scrubbed the paint off my car using the scratch remover you bought." That was the only way it would end— the only way to escape an SAF episode, the only way to avoid sleeping on the floor next to Violet and Rockwell at night.

By this point, Greyson had become so argumentative that I couldn't speak while he was around. He'd correct every word I said, even if I was talking to someone else. Correcting silly things like when I asked Michael to grab Violet's Mickey Mouse pajamas.

"They're not Mickey Mouse pajamas, they're heart pajamas," Greyson would correct because the pajamas had a heart around each Mickey.

Or I would be singing a made-up song to the kids.

"You're singing it wrong."

"I made up the song."

"It's wrong."

Once Greyson argued with me for thirty minutes over grapes. Grapes! We were at the grocery store, and the grapes were priced at $4.99 per pound and looked awful—the stems were old and brown and the grapes were wrinkled and squishy. Even though I pointed out that they were rotten and expensive, Greyson kept throwing a two-pound bag of them in my cart.

I kept taking them out. He kept putting them back. "If you want ten dollars' worth of crappy grapes, then get a job and buy them yourself."

"You're buying me these grapes."

"No, I'm not."

He screamed at me, making a huge scene in the middle of the grocery store, for what felt like hours. Over grapes!

Oh, how I've missed all those nasty stares. Thank you everyone for the reminder.

I never bought the grapes that day. I chose ten dollars over self-dignity. I slept on the floor that night.

Sometimes I'd feel trapped between a rock and a hard place. Normally, I'd just give Greyson his way to avoid an SAF episode, but there were times when doing so would put my other children in danger—like when Greyson sat on Rockwell's legs. Rockwell was sick and had fallen asleep on the couch.

"Greyson, Rockwell is sick."

"So."

"You're sitting on his legs."

"No, I'm not."

"I'm looking at you, and your butt is on top of Rockwell's legs."

Silence.

"Can you please just move over a bit?"

Silence.

"Greyson, please. Just move over a foot to the left."

Silence.

"Please."

Silence. Turned on and blared the TV.

I tried to gently pry Rockwell's legs out from under Greyson while he screamed at me. I tried to be as nice as possible because I was afraid Greyson would hurt me or, even worse, hurt Rockwell.

Michael and I knew we had to protect Violet and Rockwell, so we had to dump our house. The bad news was that it took almost two years and we lost $160,000 in equity because of the horrible housing market. Instead of getting a big check at closing, we had to *bring* a big check to closing. When it was all said and done, we had absolutely no money. We sold the house at the end of Greyson's senior year, so at least he was able to finish up high school. Barely, by the way. He spent two years acing every test, but never did a lick of homework. He even aced the ACT. When I picked him up after taking the ACT, I asked him how he did. He said, "I didn't finish," so I assumed he did poorly. I pictured him sitting there, mumbling to himself what a monumental waste of time the ACT was, while fiddling with his pencil.

He got a thirty out of thirty-six. Without finishing. Or caring.

We borrowed some money for a down payment and bought a new house. It was a perfect house because both Michael and I went from having an hour-long commute to work to having a fifteen-minute commute for me and a thirty-minute commute for Michael. That was, of course, immensely secondary to the house's large, finished, walk-out basement. The stairs that led to the basement were located behind a door in the kitchen. The basement didn't look or feel like a basement because it was fully finished and had two full-size windows and a sliding glass door that led to the backyard. It was every teenager's dream—except for us. For us, it was our dream.

SURGERY IN A STORAGE CLOSET

2012

*S*hortly after we moved, I scheduled my sweet Rockwell for surgery. I had been pushing it back and pushing it back because I was so nervous. I knew I wanted it done before I returned to work, and the clock was ticking. Rockwell needed surgery for two reasons. First, the genius doctor who delivered Rockwell completely botched his circumcision. No surprise there. His penis looked like a scared turtle hiding under its shell, sticking just the tip of its nose out. Secondly, Rockwell had a testicle that never descended. I was told that if it didn't descend by age one, then it likely never would. Rockwell was twenty months old at the time. So, basically, my boy had two strikes against him down there. Every time I would change Rockwell's diaper, Michael would say, "Dude, we've gotta get that fixed." I agreed. As much as surgery scared me, I knew I didn't want him to go through life feeling self-conscious about his penis. I could see Rockwell's college buddies calling him Uniball or Turtle Dick after a streaking shtick on campus. Plus, I was told it was a very routine surgery.

I did as much research as possible. I made multiple phone

calls, met multiple surgeons, and asked a million questions. I called some mohels, Jewish people trained in the practice of brit milah, the covenant of circumcision. One of them recommended a particular hospital, stating that their urologists had "hands made of gold from God."

The day of Rockwell's surgery, I was a complete wreck. I had an uneasy feeling because the surgeon was running behind schedule, and I could sense that he was agitated when we spoke right before the surgery. How I wish I would've trusted my gut and ran out the door.

The surgeon told us that the surgery would take about an hour, so Michael and I went for a walk. I prayed the whole time. We returned within an hour, but the lady at the front desk told us they weren't finished. Scared, I sat there watching the clock tick. Almost an additional hour later, the surgeon came out. *Oh, thank God!*

"How did it go? How's Rockwell?"

"It was fine," he said sharply in a tone I didn't like.

"Fine?"

"Yeah. It was fine," in the same tone I still didn't like.

I went to Rockwell's hospital room. It was so hard seeing my sweet baby in that state of coming out of surgery. I wished I were lying there instead.

When we arrived home, I looked at the incision on his pelvis. Hmm. . . . It was a much larger incision than I'd envisioned. It didn't look like the nice, small, clean cut I was expecting, like the one I had from my ectopic pregnancy surgery. And a two-month-old fetus had to fit through my incision. I didn't like the looks of Rockwell's incision at all. Rockwell also seemed to have an abnormally large amount of swelling, so I called the hospital.

"Hi. I was given this number when my son had surgery at your hospital today."

"Yes. How can I help you?"

"I'm concerned that my son has a lot of swelling around his incision."

"Is there a yellow or green discharge coming out of the incision?"

"No."

"Does he have a fever?"

"No."

"Swelling is expected after surgery. If it doesn't go down after a few days, give us a call."

Humph.

I hardly slept that night and kept checking his incision. I really didn't like the looks of it. I called the hospital back the next day. We literally had the exact same conversation.

And the next day.

And the next day.

And the next day. The guy answering the phone didn't like me one bit.

Maybe I was being paranoid. Rockwell was acting okay. He wasn't his usual happy self, but that was to be expected. So I decided to play it safe and take him to the pediatrician's office. She basically told me to "just keep an eye on him."

No kidding.

The days went by, and I just kept feeling like something wasn't right. Plus, the swelling hadn't gone down. It actually looked worse, or maybe it was just my imagination. I was psyching myself out. Everyone at the hospital thought I was crazy, so when I told them it looked worse they were like, "Ya sure 'bout that?"

I made another appointment with the pediatrician. On a Saturday—a very, very busy Saturday. I hadn't switched pediatricians yet, so the office was near our old house, about a thirty-minute drive. I arrived at the office and had a seat in the waiting room with about fifteen other people. I waited and waited and waited. Over two hours later, they finally called Rockwell's name. Thankfully, Rockwell had been sleeping in his carrier the entire time.

When I took Rockwell out of the carrier, his body went completely limp. He was like a dishrag—unable to even hold up his head. The pediatrician and I exchanged concerned looks, then she carefully opened his diaper and screamed. Literally screamed. Like she'd just become a doctor yesterday. When I looked at Rockwell's pelvis, I started trembling and crying hysterically.

Somehow, during those past three hours, Rockwell went from "He seems more swollen today" to "What the hell happened!?" His pelvis was discolored and enlarged to the size of a football. When I thought Rockwell was sleeping in the waiting room, he was actually dying from sepsis.

Sepsis is an extreme reaction to an infection and can worsen rapidly. Sepsis kills about 270,000 Americans each year—6 million people worldwide. In Rockwell's case, his surgical incision had become infected.

In that moment, I was too distressed and frantic to think clearly, and maybe the pediatrician was too. A good pediatrician would've called an ambulance; Rockwell's pediatrician called his surgeon. She gave me the phone, her hands visibly shaking. I started crying and screaming at him for help.

"Meet me at the hospital" he said.

I immediately ran out of her office, which was an hour away from the hospital in downtown Chicago. As I drove like a maniac, I yelled at myself for going to that pediatrician's office—thirty minutes further from Chicago than my new house. When I got closer to Chicago, the traffic was horrible. Cars were lined up bumper to bumper, and I was still several miles away. I got on the shoulder of the expressway and drove for miles, passing all the still cars, bawling so uncontrollably I was having trouble seeing the road. People were honking and yelling at me out their windows. I was so afraid Rockwell wouldn't make it to the hospital. I kept looking in my rearview mirror—which I had adjusted to look at Rockwell instead of the road—yelling his name every few minutes to check for signs of life.

I pulled up and saw Rockwell's surgeon waiting for me outside. I illegally parked at the front of the hospital. He led us into a small room about twenty feet from the entrance. It looked like a storage closet, furnished with only a bench and shelves of medical supplies. He snapped at a random nurse to get him surgical scissors and some kind of medical gauze. He placed Rockwell on the bench and manually opened his wound. The surgeon then took a jar full of what looked like about eighteen inches of half-inch-thick, moistened, medical gauze and slowly inserted it into Rockwell's now-opened wound. Rockwell just laid there—lifelessly—seemingly unaware that his wound was split open and over a foot of gauze was stuffed into his body. The surgeon then closed up his wound, leaving a few inches of the gauze hanging out. "Slowly pull this out tomorrow morning," he instructed me.

Did my son just have emergency surgery in a storage closet?

That was the worst day of my life.

I have never, ever been so frightened as I was that day. I almost lost my Rockwell. I almost lost my buddy . . . my pal. As I sit here and write, Rockwell is now eight years old. It took me weeks to write this chapter because it's so painful. I've thought about that horrific day every day since it happened, but writing about it was excruciating. Rockwell is now in second grade, and just like I knew the first moment I held him, he's the coolest kid on the planet. He's in a good mood every single day and has the greatest sense of humor. A keen humor I've never witnessed in a child, even though I've taught children near his age for two decades. Rockwell gets straight As and his teachers describe him as very smart, well liked, and mature. He is very sensitive and conscientious of other people's feelings. Rockwell is an amazing golfer and wins first place in almost every tournament he enters. His best score so far was a thirty-five for nine holes—he beat eighteen-year-old golfers in the same tournament. His favorite game is chess, and his favorite foods are lobster and escargot. He loves classical music and Elvis Presley. Rockwell is gorgeous, a half foot taller than his classmates, and he inherited my grandfather's barrel chest. If I could've created a wish list of everything I'd want my son to be, I couldn't have possibly come up with all the wonderful things that he is. And I almost lost him from a "routine" surgery. I almost lost him because no one seemed to care. I almost lost him because medical professionals don't always listen. I almost lost him because I didn't trust my instincts.

But I thank God every day that I didn't lose him. Violet still has her best friend. Michael still has his beloved son and golf buddy. My parents still have a grandson to spoil who never acts spoiled. I still have a son who runs to hug me when I get home from work and makes me laugh every single day.

But for now, returning to my story, Rockwell wasn't even two and my sweet girl was only three. And, more than anything, I had to protect Violet and Rockwell. I had to protect them more within the four walls of my home than from the sometimes cruel world. Because the year Greyson was seventeen was the year my light for him went dim. The boy who I'd wholeheartedly believed would do something spectacular in this world had become the boy I fretted would do something inconceivable in this world. When Greyson was seventeen, his behavior had become so bizarre and so severe so rapidly that I began to think of his childhood as the easy years.

Before we'd moved, which was immediately after

Greyson graduated from high school, I'd taken one last look at that shampoo bottle sitting in Greyson's shower. That little Sharpie mark haunted me for months as I checked it daily praying each time the shampoo would fall below that line. But it didn't. That damn shampoo stayed right at that damn line. My heart sank every time I looked. If my math was correct, Greyson hadn't washed his hair in almost a year. He turned the shower on every day, got his hair wet every day, but he never washed it. It appeared he also hadn't combed his hair in a year because it was matted. Greyson refused to step out of the car when I pulled up to a hair salon, so it also hadn't been cut in a year.

I had also been keeping an eye on other hygiene products like his soap and toothpaste. I noticed those were never used either. Greyson's teeth started to look gray. When he spoke, I stared at his teeth and could see a film so thick there was a visible indentation where his lips normally rested.

In addition, Greyson no longer bothered to change his clothes. He had a dresser full of clothes that just sat there untouched. He wouldn't change his outfit for months—not even at bedtime. When I offered to wash his outfit, he screamed at me.

Greyson also stopped using deodorant. Needless to say, his body odor became so intolerable that it was difficult being in the same room as him. I tried talking to him about my concerns, but, as usual, those words fell on deaf ears.

As we got settled into our three-bedroom, ranch-style home, Greyson moved into his huge, fully finished, walk-out basement. Our old house had been nearly 4,000 square feet, while our new home was only 1,500 square feet, so we had a lot of extra furniture. Since the basement was as big as the rest of the house, Greyson's bedroom set and all our former family room furniture fit comfortably in the basement. The separate living areas made Greyson's space feel like a cozy apartment. Making the basement really nice for him helped diminish the guilt I felt for having him live on a separate floor. Although that arrangement did reduce interaction with Greyson, it didn't completely alleviate it. The basement didn't have a kitchen or a bathroom, so he still had to come upstairs. And every day when he came upstairs, Michael and I put on our fake smiles, tried engaging him in fake conversation, and asked him to join us for dinner with fake enthusiasm. Sometimes he did join us for dinner when I served something he deemed acceptable.

Greyson's list of acceptable dinners could fit on a Post-it note. Over the past year, Greyson's diet had evolved to strictly organic, non-GMO foods. I primarily bought organic fruits, vegetables, milk, and meat, but I also had a pantry full of nonorganic items. If I so much as seasoned with a nonorganic seasoning or buttered vegetables with a nonorganic butter or even sprayed the pan with a nonorganic cooking spray, Greyson wouldn't eat what I'd made. He went from loving my cooking to hardly touching it. *Just for the record, I make kickass steak and ribs.* For Greyson's sixteenth birthday, his dinner request was ribs. A year later, he wouldn't touch them. The silver lining was that Greyson would often cook his own meals. I had to turn off the stove and clean up his mess, but he did cook.

Michael and I tried with all our might not to show it, but we were on pins and needles when Greyson came upstairs. When Greyson rejected our conversations and dinner invitations and closed that basement door behind him, we would breathe a collective sigh of relief.

When we moved into our new place, I immediately put two things on the basement door: a lock and a bell. We told Greyson that the lock was there when we bought the house and the bell was there to let us know if Violet or Rockwell went near the stairs (even though we also had a baby gate guarding the basement door). Greyson accepted my explanation knowing how protective I was.

At first, we never locked the basement door because Greyson came upstairs many times throughout the day to cook, use the restroom, and "shower." Michael slept on the couch every night so he could hear the bell if it rang. Each morning I'd ask Michael if Greyson had come up in the middle of the night, and each morning, Michael said no. It seemed odd that Greyson never once used the restroom in the middle of the night.

"Hey Greyson, do you ever need to use the restroom in the middle of the night?"

"No."

"Rockwell is at the stage where he can climb out of his crib and over this gate. Would it be okay if we locked the basement door before we went to bed at night? We can unlock it when we get up at six."

"Fine."

"Are you sure? What if you have to use the restroom?"

"I won't."

"Okay, thanks. Let me know if you change your mind. You can always knock on the door if you have to go."

From that moment on, Michael and I slept a little better at night, knowing that door was locked.

A HELLACIOUS ROAD TO NOWHERE

2012–2014

I confided in my aunt about the difficulties I was having with Greyson. This was the same aunt I'd lived near in Minnesota back when Greyson was four years old—the same aunt who'd performed the ceremony when Michael and I were married. I felt my aunt was a good person to talk to because she had a doctorate in theology and was a Baptist minister at a church she'd founded for the homeless. Basically, she's a saint. She offered to take Greyson for a few months hoping she could help guide him. She thought perhaps Greyson getting away would help him find himself, clear his mind, or reflect on his life. *I'll take D. All of the above, please.* I thought if anyone on this planet could help Greyson, it was my aunt.

I got Greyson a one-way train ticket to Minnesota and off he went. *Can I get a woo-hoo!?*

It was so nice to finally feel relaxed in my home. I stopped worrying every time the bell on the basement door jiggled. I stopped worrying every time I left Violet and Rockwell alone in the family room for a moment. I stopped worrying about what Greyson was really doing in the basement when he didn't come upstairs at his usual time. For the first time in a long time, I felt safe.

For ten days.

Not ten business days.

Just ten actual days.

Two hundred forty hours of bliss.

That's how long my aunt lasted.

It wasn't her fault. She gave it a good go. She took Greyson fishing, they went to the farmers market, they worked in her garden—all things Greyson typically enjoyed. She even took Greyson to chop wood. *Yikes*. Greyson loved it, but the idea of him holding an ax sent shivers down my spine.

Still, after ten days, my aunt put Greyson on a plane back to Chicago. She said Greyson threatened her, and she refused to be afraid in her own home. *Sounds about right.* Clearly, she'd experienced one of Greyson's SAF episodes, and I called them Scary as Fuck for a reason. At least I learned that Michael and I weren't crazy for being scared of Greyson. My aunt blamed Greyson's behavior on what she believed to be "untreated Asperger's syndrome." I could see why she thought that. I never mentioned to her that Greyson had been in therapy on and off throughout his life. More off than on, though, because the six or so different therapists I'd tried never seemed to help—even my favorite one, who saw Greyson every week for about a year. He was delightful, but I never noticed any change in Greyson. Plus, in all honesty, those therapists never told me anything I didn't already know.

When Greyson was sixteen, he had seen two different therapists. They added depression and Asperger's syndrome to Greyson's laundry list of diagnoses. The term *Asperger's syndrome* is often used interchangeably with high-functioning autism, but in 1994, the *Diagnostic and Statistical*

Manual of Mental Disorders (DSM) began listing them as separate disorders. Then in 2013, the *DSM* took all subcategories and put them under one umbrella diagnosis of autism spectrum disorder (ASD). Greyson was diagnosed with Asperger's syndrome in 2010, a few years before this change. Since different doctors often give different clinical diagnoses, Greyson was technically diagnosed with both disorders.

Over the years, Greyson had been given a lot of different diagnoses but never any strategies or solutions that worked. Greyson even tried a few different meds, but the side effects were always too severe, or so he said. Eventually, Greyson refused therapy. I'd drive him there, persuading him with Panda Express (his fave spot before going organic), but when we'd arrive at the therapist's office, he'd refuse to get out of the car. I did that at least five times before giving up.

So, yes, I suppose my aunt was correct in saying Greyson had untreated Asperger's.

And autism.

And depression.

And oppositional defiant disorder.

And sensory processing disorder.

I alphabetized them for your ease-of-viewing pleasure. The only thing my aunt e-mailed me that I found bothersome was, "You have the power. You have the power to take a course on Asperger's to help you develop strategies on how to help Greyson."

My aunt can now add comedian to her credentials. She does realize I have a master's degree in education, correct? Pretty sure that was mentioned in one of my parents' Christmas cards.

Maybe it wasn't obvious that I had to take child psychology classes while earning my bachelor's and master's degrees in education. I've also attended countless workshops, seminars, and professional development sessions relating to children with disabilities, which is required at my job as a teacher at an all-inclusive school where, each year, one-fourth of my students had some form of disability. I felt like saying, "I'm actually qualified to teach the class you're recommending I attend."

Most people believe that both environment and genetics influence behavior. I agree. However, before I had Greyson, I believed personalities were formed 90 percent from environmental factors and 10 percent from biological factors. Now, having raised both mentally ill and "normal" children, I believe personalities are formed 90 percent from biological factors and 10 percent from environmental factors. (Like with most things in life, there are exceptions. Personality traits may be altered due to extreme conditions in environmental factors, such as someone who has endured emotional, physical, or sexual abuse.)

Had I never raised Greyson, I'd likely still believe that environment is the primary contributing factor in a child's personality, success, or failure. I would probably think that Violet and Rockwell have straight As and beautiful behavior because I'm just that amazing of a mom. I'd walk out of Violet and Rockwell's parent-teacher conferences and think, *Wow, I sure have my shit together.* I'd judge my friends with the naughty kids and think, *I really should give them some advice since I've got this parenting thing down.* But because I have raised Greyson, when a parent cries during parent-teacher conferences and says, "I'm not sure why Johnny acts this way; his siblings aren't like this," I am empathetic, and I understand. I'm a very good listener, but I don't dare mention Greyson.

I stopped talking about Greyson when my joy turned into sadness.

I stopped talking about Greyson when my pride turned into fear.

I stopped talking about Greyson when my dreams turned into heartbreak.

Yes, those were the years I stopped talking about Greyson to every human being.

Little by little, I stopped talking about Greyson to my friends. When friends would come over and see Greyson, I could sense their pity. It's just human nature to see a long-haired, dirty-clothed, gray-toothed, foul-smelling, back-talking son and wonder what I did wrong. (Except Molly, she knew me too well to think that.) I imagined what they'd think if my friends went into the basement. Greyson had started leaving half-eaten fruit, uneaten meals, and piles of trash all over the furniture and the floor. Despite his six-foot-five frame, Greyson weighed only 120 pounds because he would only take a few bites of food then leave it out to rot. If my friends went into the basement, they'd see thirty jugs of water on the floor that Greyson had filtered with the $300 filtration system I had to buy so he would drink. Greyson no longer trusted water unless he'd filtered it himself. In fact, he'd gotten to the point where he wouldn't even rinse off in the shower. If my friends snooped in the basement, they'd find an additional fifty gallons of water Greyson had hidden in the walls behind our water meter and piping to "prepare him for terrorism or a natural disaster."

Little by little, I stopped talking about Greyson to my relatives. Actually, none of my relatives knew much about Greyson because they were scattered all over the country. I'd have small talk and brag about Greyson with relatives a couple times a year over the phone, and they'd all read about Greyson's academic achievements in my parents' Christmas cards. Of course I never mentioned, and my parents never wrote, about all my struggles over the years. That wouldn't make for a very joyous Christmas card. But when I did periodically talk to them, what could I say? That I found an ax and a baseball bat hidden in Greyson's basement apartment? Or that Greyson signed up to volunteer at an organic farm but got sent home his second day because the farmer was afraid to have him in her home.

Little by little, I stopped talking about Greyson on Facebook. In the past, I'd occasionally post a proud video of Greyson playing the drums or a picture of Greyson holding his baby brother or sister. But now what could I post? I certainly couldn't post a picture of him. I couldn't ask my Facebook friends to join Greyson in his movement to abolish money. Greyson now believed there was no need for money in society and that it would soon no longer exist. Greyson actually believed individuals would go back to trading services and products so the exchange of currency would no longer be needed. Maybe I could've posted that Greyson cured cancer. He did, you know. He wholeheartedly believed that he'd found a cure for cancer in our basement.

Little by little, I stopped talking about Greyson to my sister. Well, actually, I'd stopped talking to her about Greyson when he was a baby. I learned very early on that even though I only saw my sister two or three times a year, she dissected every move I made and every word I said—so much so that I hadn't acted myself around her since I was a teenager. There was no one who knew me less in the world yet thought she knew me the most. When I was little, I listened to my sister more than anyone in the world, but I couldn't listen to parenting advice from someone who'd never been a parent. She thought she was an expert on child-rearing because she had a dog. I wondered what my sister would've said if I told her Greyson had covered all his windows and mirrors with black garbage bags. She'd probably say he had a poor self-image. I wondered what my sister would've said if I told her Greyson never used the bathroom because he urinated in jars, put his bowel movements in Ziploc bags, and never used toilet paper. She'd probably say I'd potty trained him too early. One thing was for certain—in her eyes, it was all my fault.

Little by little, I stopped talking about Greyson to my parents. That was difficult. My parents loved Greyson so much, and I didn't want to break their hearts. Like me for so long, they could only see Greyson's strengths. Like me for so long, they believed Greyson had a bright future. Like me for so long, they were proud of Greyson. Although, eventually, my parents' joy, pride, and dreams fizzled like mine, but they sure fought a good fight. They tried so hard to turn a blind eye to Greyson's behaviors. But they couldn't ignore it when Greyson stole a hundred dollars from my mom's purse. They couldn't ignore it when Greyson told my mom to shut up while she was moaning in pain during a severe gout attack. They couldn't ignore it when Greyson pushed them when they tried to hug him. We could no longer collaboratively pretend Greyson was our crowning achievement.

Little by little, I stopped talking about Greyson to his coworkers who tried to help him. Yes, Greyson had a job—a job at the organic store he frequented for all his organic food and products. He'd been such a good customer—often educating the employees about the benefits of each herbal supplement. The store manager had good intentions when she decided to employ an autistic young man. Little did the manager know that Greyson would steal $2,000 worth of food and products before getting fired. At least Greyson didn't deposit his paychecks. I'd find them scrunched in a ball, full of dirt and rips on the floor of the basement. He received paper paychecks because he refused to fill out the half-page document for direct deposit.

One of Greyson's coworkers, a fifty-five-year-old woman

and mother of four adult boys, approached me to point out that Greyson needed help. *Really? I had no idea.* She offered to take Greyson in, as if I weren't doing my job as a mother. I chuckled to myself at her naivety and looked forward to a couple days of peace in my home. She lasted a week, which was actually six days longer than I'd expected. Then she called me and said, "Come get your son right now, this instant. I'm fearful for my life." She told me she was going to file a restraining order against him.

Little by little, I stopped talking about Greyson to the teachers at my school. Before my maternity leave, I'd share good news about Greyson, like all good moms do. I'd tell them when Greyson got straight As or when he'd received another academic award or was accepted into another gifted program. I'd beam with pride when I spoke about Greyson. But at this point, what could I say? That Greyson stayed up every night, all night long, then slept all day. That Greyson wasn't going to college and had no future goals. My coworkers often asked with such enthusiasm and genuineness how Greyson was doing. My answers became so vague, "He's great!" I'd say. If they only knew what was going through my mind on that horrific day in December 2012, when several teachers received alerts on their phones at lunchtime, "Mass school shooting at Sandy Hook Elementary School." Not knowing where Sandy Hook was, I frantically ran to look at my friend's alert. "When? Just now? Where? Near here? Who did it?" My body shook, my voice trembled, I felt ill. Those endless three minutes when I didn't have more information, all I kept thinking was, *Please don't let Greyson be the shooter. Please don't let Greyson be the shooter. Please don't let Greyson be the shooter.*

Little by little, I stopped talking about Greyson to psychologists; I had given up on them when Greyson was sixteen. But with his recent incomprehensible behaviors, I was desperate. I spent hours calling every psychologist in the area looking for someone—anyone—who specialized in treating people like Greyson—if there *was* anyone like Greyson. I finally made an appointment, but when I drove him there, Greyson wouldn't get out of the car. I begged him and begged him, telling him I just wanted to help. He finally got out of the car and ran into the large, four-story, office building. I ran after him, but he was nowhere to be found. I walked up and down the hallways on every floor, opening every single office door and calling his name. I eventually found him an hour later and miraculously got him to go into the psychologist's office. By then, we were extremely late, but I had stopped in at our appointment time to tell them the situation. However, Greyson refused to sign the sheet of paper required to see the psychologist, and because he was over eighteen, there was nothing I could do about it. By this time, it was dark outside and the office staff was winding down for the day. As we sat in that waiting room, the only thing that could be heard was my voice. But no matter what I said or how much I begged, I couldn't get Greyson to sign that sheet of paper.

Little by little, I stopped talking about Greyson to my neighbors. I often wondered if they saw Greyson when he walked outside wearing only ragged, stained-covered jeans in zero-degree temperatures, barefoot on the snow-covered ground. I wondered if they could tell from their bedroom windows that Greyson hadn't used soap, washed his hair, or brushed his teeth in over two years. I wondered if they noticed that Greyson couldn't drive. The car we had for Greyson became Michael's transportation to the train station for work. I wondered if they saw every time the police came to our house.

Little by little, I stopped talking about Greyson to police officers. At first I called the nonemergency number at least ten times. I wanted a documented trail of calls stating my concerns about Greyson in case something happened to us. When Greyson's episodes escalated from Scary as Fuck to Petrifying as Fuck, I started calling 911. The first few times I called 911 were similar—I blocked the entryway to the family room where Violet and Rockwell were playing while Greyson stood in a threatening stance, his fists tightly clenched. He'd scream at me relentlessly with his voice trembling, body shaking, face red with anger, and eyes rolled back showing almost only white. Every time the police came, I'd privately asked an officer, "What should I do?" or "Where can I get help?" I begged the officers to search my house for homemade explosive devices. They did once—for five minutes. I begged the officers to take Greyson's computer and search his history. I told them I was scared of Greyson. I was scared for my younger children. I was scared for other people's children. But they never helped me. They just warned me that it was against the law to kick Greyson out of the house, even though he was over eighteen. They said I must go through a legal eviction process and give him a ninety-day warning since he'd never physically harmed anyone. *Thanks dude. Superhelpful as usual.* The last time I called 911 was from a parking lot the night Greyson was kicked out of his coworker's house. Greyson was standing in the middle of the parking lot, late at night, snow heavily falling, wearing only jeans and a T-shirt. There was a jacket I didn't recognize lying next to him on the ground. He kept yelling at me that he didn't do anything wrong—that his coworker had kicked him out of her house for no reason. I tried hugging him to calm him down and get him warm. Then he screamed that I'd put something on his back when I hugged him. He took off his T-shirt to make sure nothing was there, then tossed it on the snow-covered ground next to the mystery jacket. Then he knelt on the freezing ground in the middle of the dimly lit parking lot now wearing only jeans. He wouldn't stand up. He wouldn't get dressed. He wouldn't get in the car. He wouldn't stop yelling that he didn't do anything wrong. When the police arrived, they searched his jeans, his snow-covered shirt, and the mystery jacket where they found a pipe in the pocket—no drugs, just a pipe. Even though Greyson explained it was his coworker's jacket, which was true, they gave him a $500 ticket. Or should I say they gave *me* a $500 ticket since I'm the one who paid it. And with lawyer fees, it actually turned into a $2,000 ticket. *Thanks police officers. Could've done without that.* The only thing the police did do—that should've been helpful, but wasn't—was send Greyson to mental health hospitals.

Little by little, I stopped talking about Greyson to mental health hospitals. The first time the police sent Greyson to a mental health hospital, he was taken in an ambulance, tested for drugs, and kept overnight. The drug tests, as usual, came back negative. The second time, I lied to the police. I had found out that by merely using the correct terminology, Greyson would go to the mental health hospital for three days instead of one. So I said, "Greyson lifted his arm to hit me." I thought that was the only way I could get Greyson seen by multiple doctors and psychologists. But when Greyson returned home three days later, it was like he'd never went. Well, except for the thousands of dollars in bills I received for the ambulance rides, doctor visits, and hospital stays. Even so, the third time, I lied to the police again. I was desperate for Greyson to see more doctors and psychologists, hopefully better ones that time. Plus, I'd get three days of feeling safe in my home. The last time he went, Greyson went to the "best" hospital in the area where we knew an employee. That employee pulled some strings for us, and Greyson stayed for a week. Still, when he returned home, nothing had changed—except our bank account. Even though we had insurance, I received a mountain of bills for thousands and thousands and thousands of dollars—a separate bill for every test given, every doctor seen, and every night he stayed. Still, no one offered any solutions for what to do outside those hospital walls. Greyson did, however, receive more diagnoses (from multiple hospitals) to add to his growing list: schizophrenia and schizoaffective disorder.

Schizoaffective disorder and schizophrenia are both psychotic disorders that include symptoms of delusions (false beliefs), hallucinations (hearing, seeing, or feeling things that aren't there), and disorganized thinking. With both conditions, symptoms tend to surface between the late teens and early twenties for men. However, new research has detected schizophrenia in the womb, suggesting that it's an unwanted side effect during the development of the brain, particularly when pregnant mothers experience high levels of stress. Schizoaffective disorder is a combination of both schizophrenia and a mood disorder, such as bipolar disorder (mania and major depression) or depressive disorder (major depression without mania). Greyson was diagnosed with schizophrenia then bipolar, which ultimately resulted in a schizoaffective disorder diagnosis, totaling eight diagnoses thus far.

Little by little, I stopped talking about Greyson to other professionals who were supposedly there to help. I had tried at one of my recent teacher workshops. The workshop was about how to handle bullies. After the workshop, I approached the speaker because he'd mentioned some services and help centers for teenagers that I thought might be able to help Greyson. During my inquiries, the speaker kept asking me questions to get more information to "help" me. When I hesitantly revealed I was actually inquiring about my own son, he blamed me for raising a bully. He spoke to me as if I were a criminal. As if my poor parenting skills were counterproductive to his war against bullies. Instead of leaving with information, I left feeling bullied.

Little by little, I stopped talking about Greyson to government offices. We were spending thousands and thousands and thousands of dollars on Greyson. Thousands of dollars on Greyson's medical bills. Thousands of dollars on Greyson's lawyer fees. Thousands of dollars meeting all Greyson's demands like his filtration system, his organic futon, and his hyperorganic diet and supplements. Thousands of dollars on property Greyson was destroying in our home. When Greyson destroyed our carpet, video camera, lawn mower, and the paint on my car, that was just the beginning. He also destroyed all our family room furniture, his mattresses, our lawn chairs, Michael's bike, the list went on and on. We had to use every cent of both our paychecks each month and all of Greyson's college savings just to scratch the surface of Greyson's bills. I knew Greyson must qualify for government assistance, but Greyson refused to go to the government offices with me to sign the paperwork. I kept calling and calling and calling different government offices trying to get help—any help at all—but everyone said Greyson had to come in to sign the paperwork. "May I ask, how I'm supposed to get a six-foot-five-inch man with Asperger's, autism, depression, oppositional defiant disorder, sensory processing disorder, and schizoaffective disorder into an office to sign a sheet of paper? I can't even get him to use the toilet." I even called the FBI once—on the day Greyson said to me, "I'm going to show you that everyone is wrong. I'm going to show the world that everyone is wrong." His tone sent shivers down my spine. The look in his eyes as he spoke was the look of a killer. I called the FBI and told them what he said. I told them Greyson had every warning sign of a mass murderer. I begged them to tap into or take his computer to look for signs. I asked them to search my house. The woman on the other line hung up on me.

Little by little, I stopped talking about Greyson to mental health treatment centers. I called what seemed like every mental health treatment center in the country. I created spreadsheets comparing and contrasting them. I took notes upon notes upon notes that I kept in my "Mental Health Treatment Center" notebook—not to be confused with my "Government Offices" notebook or my "Mental Institutions and Doctors" notebook. But the holistic mental health treatment centers that Greyson found acceptable were astronomically expensive, and the reasonably priced options, he refused. Plus, he was over eighteen, so by law, I couldn't force him into treatment.

Little by little, I stopped talking about Greyson to Michael. After all, Michael had been right about Greyson: he was a nightmare, although he never could've predicted things would be this bad. Michael and I had nothing left to say. By that time, all we did was live in fear that Greyson might hurt Violet and Rockwell. Greyson had already accidentally fractured Violet's wrist when he yanked on her arm. Greyson had already almost blinded Rockwell when he told Rockwell to jump into his arms then didn't catch him. Rockwell landed face-first into the tip of his rocking horse. The doctors told us how lucky we were, "Another millimeter to the right, and he'd be blind in one eye."

Little by little, I stopped talking about Greyson to Greyson. By the time he was nineteen, my attempts at conversation with him were either met with long silences then one-word exchanges or overly elaborate circular conversations that I couldn't escape. Greyson would go on and on about how his cavity fillings were slowly killing him and that he called several dentists asking if they could remove his fillings but not replace them. He insisted that when two of his fillings fell out, he started feeling much better and that he was willing to go to Mexico to have the rest removed. He talked about how exercise was bad for you and how it was healthy to exude the most minimal amount of energy possible. He talked about all the remedies he'd discovered—for gastritis it was flexing your muscles, shaking, and squinting your face. If I said anything disputing his opinions, he'd say, "You're being rhetorical and have no standpoints," or "You're an evil spirit and a parasite."

Little by little, I stopped talking about Greyson—after almost two solid years of only talking about him. Those were the years I functioned on a level of hysterics and desperation. Those were the years I spent anywhere from ten to twenty hours a week making phone calls seeking some sort of help for Greyson—all while caring for two young children and working full-time. Most doctors, psychologists, mental health treatment centers, and government offices were only open Monday through Friday. I used all thirty of my sick and personal days those two years just to stay home and make phone calls seeking help for Greyson. Once my fifteen sick and personal days per year were gone, I had no choice but to make calls from work. I'd dial a number, put the handset on my desk with the speaker volume very low, elevator music playing in the background, and sometimes wait on hold for over an hour at a time, all while teaching first grade. I got really good at teaching while paying just enough attention to the phone so when a person finally picked up, I'd run to my desk yelling, "I'm here! I'm here! I'm here! Don't hang up!" The secretary at my school, who I adored, kept my secret. She didn't know exactly what was going on, but I often went to the front office, tail between my legs and said, "Um, I'm waiting for another call (from this doctor, this treatment center, or this office), so could you please put them through to my classroom, not to my voice mail?" Understandably, teachers were not supposed to be on the phone while teaching, so calls normally got directed to voice mail. The secretary would give me a sympathetic smile and a nod. She never questioned me. We'd been working together for almost a decade, and she knew I was a dedicated teacher. She knew something was very wrong because I would never talk on the phone while teaching unless it was critical.

Still, all my efforts, all my desperate cries for help, every effort and cry, every cry and effort, just led to dead ends.

I felt hopeless.

Exhausted.

Defeated.

Lost.

During those two years, every single night before I went to bed, I took each stool from the island in our kitchen, and one by one, I silently, painstakingly, stacked them up against the basement door. I no longer trusted just a jiggle to wake us up. I no longer trusted that ten-dollar lock.

Those two years, every single morning when I woke up, I silently, painstakingly, took the stools down, one by one, and returned them to the island hoping Greyson would never find out.

Then every single morning when I left for work, I grabbed my essential coffee, my to-do call list, and my three dreadful notebooks.

Those two years, every single day and every single night, I prayed Greyson wouldn't kill us.

HUMANS WITH COMMON SENSE
NEED NOT APPLY

2014–2015

My entire life, I've been very healthy. I'm told I look young for my age. In addition to genetics, I assume it's because I eat well and take care of myself. I've always been active and thin. Yes, I'm a foodie. I love a good steak, a deep-dish Chicago–style pizza, and homemade cookies, but I've always been good about eating unhealthy foods in moderation. I crave fruits and vegetables. I rarely eat anything fried. I can go years between fast-food visits. I drink very little alcohol and soda. However, in 2014, a few months before Greyson's twentieth birthday, I turned into a medical wreck—a giant ball of stress mess.

For the past three years, since Greyson had turned seventeen, I'd experienced immense panic attacks on a daily basis. I used to get panic attacks when Greyson was young, during those years when he beat me, but they'd gone away. But at this point, my panic attacks had become so severe that my doctors ran a series of tests on my heart. My heartbeat often felt so weak that I couldn't feel it through my chest. I had to sit silently, perfectly still, with my fingers placed on my wrist or on my throat just to locate the faintest heartbeat. Sometimes I never did feel it, but I thought, *Well, it must be beating—barely.* Sometimes my heartbeat fluttered, which made me feel disoriented. Other times, I had to sit and concentrate on breathing as lightly as possible because each inhale sent a shooting pain to my chest.

I often had intense stomach pain too. I would lay on the floor curled up in a ball unable to stand or even sit upright. I had to just lay there and wait for the pain to subside. There were times when I was out and Michael had to come pick me up because I was in too much pain to drive. At school, there were days when the speech pathologist had to temporarily cover my class.

I also had terrible residual effects from the horrific epidural that caused me to have Bell's palsy. My legs were sometimes wobbly. My teeth didn't line up correctly when I chewed or spoke. My speech slurred. My toes went numb. It would come and go, but it worsened under stress, which was nonstop during that time. Those symptoms led to a series of tests including an MRI of my brain—twice. To this day, I still suffer from these symptoms—as well as others—and they've become even worse over time. The doctors don't believe me when I blame my epidural, even though they don't have any answers. Even though it all started the moment that needle went into my spine. Stay tuned for my next book, *Doctors Ruin Lives.*

I couldn't take it anymore. I couldn't take the stress of Greyson while raising two young children and working full-time. I felt like a prisoner in my own home and in my body. I'd finally reached my breaking point.

Physically.

Emotionally.

Psychologically.

Financially.

I.

Could.

Not.

Take.

One.

More.

Day.

I kicked Greyson out of the house.

He took his laptop and the clothes on his back. I gave him all my cash.

Fuck every police officer who told me I couldn't.

Fuck every relative who told me I shouldn't.

Fuck every person I pleaded to for help.

Fuck every doctor I paid for no reason.

Fuck the government and its stupid red tape.

Fuck Sperm Donor who was "in a relationship" with a pretty twenty-six-year-old.

Fuck Facebook for showing me that.

Ya know what? Just fuck the whole fucking world.

Do you have a problem with me kicking him out? I thought not.

Greyson joined a couch-surfing website and stayed in strangers' homes. I never knew that existed. Strangers just let him stay in their homes—for free. Can you believe that's a thing? It's like hitchhiking but for a place to sleep. Each night he had to find a different couch. I'm not sure if that was a couch-surfing policy or a just-met-Greyson-in-person policy.

When Greyson wasn't couch-surfing, he stayed at a hostel in Chicago. I met Greyson once a week to give him cash so he could survive. He told me he sometimes begged for money on the streets. I couldn't give Greyson too much cash at once because I knew it was inevitable that he'd lose some of it. I evenly divided the cash among his four jean pockets so he was less likely to lose it all at once.

This went on for over a month. During that time, I replaced my dreadful notebooks with a new dreadful notebook. This one was titled "Housing." Sounds so simple, right? Not so much. Trying to find affordable housing for Greyson was extremely challenging because Greyson loved making everything challenging. That notebook had lots of tabs—color-coded tabs that I thought made sense. There was the "Transitional Housing Programs" tab, the "Homeless Youth Programs" tab, the "Christian Housing Programs" tab, and the "YMCA Housing Programs" tab. Every type of housing that offered some sort of support, counseling, or subsidized rent had a tab. Tab, tab, tab, tab. Then there were the tabs that Greyson thought made sense, including the "Organic Farm Housing" tab, the "Apartments" tab, and the "Rooms for Rent Through Craigslist" tab.

I did all the research. I made all the calls. And I took all the notes. Research. Calls. Notes. Research. Calls. Notes. I did over a month of research, calls, and notes. I must've found fifty reasonable options for Greyson all over the country. I looked in other states more than I looked in Illinois. Just because Greyson was out of our house didn't mean we weren't still scared. He knew where we lived.

Every option I suggested, he'd say no. And he'd say no. And he'd say no. And he'd say no, no, no, no. I felt I was approaching insanity because I must have done a hundred hours of research, calls, and notes knowing full well that Greyson would never accept any of them. Again, and I can't stress this enough, *according to the law*, I could not make Greyson do anything. Even when I knew it was in his best interest. Even though common sense told me my foul-smelling, six-foot-five-inch, 120-pound son needed medical help, I could not make him go to a doctor.

Even though common sense told me my voice-hearing,

hallucination-seeing, schizoaffective son needed a prescription, I could not make him swallow a pill.

Even though common sense told me my film-covered, gray-toothed son needed dental help, I could not make him go to a dentist.

Even though common sense told me my penniless, destitute son qualified for financial assistance, free medical insurance, and a free cell phone, I could not make him walk into a government office to sign a sheet of paper so he would stop draining our bank account.

Even though common sense told me my mentally incapable, psychologically disturbed son qualified to live in subsidized housing that offered counseling and support, I could not make him live in housing where he'd be safe.

Even though I'm chock-full of all this common sense, *according to the law*, I could not help my son.

After over a month of me pounding my head against a brick wall, or so it felt, Greyson found an apartment through Craigslist. In Tennessee. With a roommate. Whom he knew nothing about.

Of course, I knew that was a bad idea. Of course, I stated my opinion to Greyson. Of course, I spoke to Greyson's middle-aged, soon-to-be roommate and warned him that Greyson had multiple diagnoses and that I'd kicked him out of the house. But neither of them flinched when I gave my opinion.

So off Greyson went.

Who paid for his security deposit? His rent? His cell phone? His organic blanket? His organic pillow? His organic food? The glass jars that he used interchangeably for food and piss? Well, Michael and me of course!

That living arrangement was short-lived.

And so was the next.

And the next.

And the next.

And he never packed, he just left everything behind.

Let's just throw it all on top of the thousands and thousands and thousands of dollars in bills we were already drowning in from Greyson—the rotten cherry on top of a melted sundae, if you will.

CALIFORNIA DREAMIN'

2015

*A*fter enduring years of absolute hell, Michael and I made a rash decision to move to California. I think we wanted to get as far away as possible from the last five years of our lives. We chose California because my parents lived there, and we were very close to them. We were also sick of Chicago weather that could dip down to negative forty degrees with the windchill factored in. And sadly, just the thought of Greyson showing up at our doorstep terrified us.

It was very difficult leaving my best friend, Molly, but her husband was applying for positions in Washington, DC, at the time, so they were preparing for a new life on the opposite end of the country from where we'd decided to start ours. They left Chicago shortly after us, but Molly and I talked almost every day.

It took me two months to hand in my letter of resignation at work, even though I had told my principal I was moving. Saying goodbye to my job and teacher friends was the hardest part about leaving Chicago. I'd been at the same school for a decade. I loved that job and my coworkers were the best. We always had so much fun in the teachers' lounge. Every day, we'd laugh so hard that we cried.

The staff threw me a surprise farewell party. The librarian and principal got up in front of the entire staff and performed a song and dance for me. It was so hilarious and adorable. Imagine two brilliant, conservative, professional women wearing matching outfits, dancing, and singing a song they wrote about me to the tune of "California Dreamin'." That was the nicest thing anyone had ever done for me. I tear up just thinking about how much I miss that job and those women.

So off we went to Southern California. We moved into a temporary apartment, and I immediately applied for teaching jobs. I was pleased to get multiple offers. I chose the second grade position closest to where we were shopping for a new home. We qualified to buy a new home because I'd signed a teaching contract and Michael was working remotely for his employer back in Chicago. We were also able to pay off our mountain of Greyson debt when we sold our house in Chicago for a great price.

I was so excited to start my new teaching job—excited to make new friends, excited to wow my new principal and parents, excited to no longer live in fear, excited to finally be Claire.

My new principal was too young to have much teaching experience. She was tall, beautiful, slender, and dressed like a million bucks—designer shoes, designer clothes, every bleach blonde hair in place. Principal Barbie had a permanent fake smile plastered on her face and a sickeningly cheery voice.

Next, there was the Wicked Witch of the West, otherwise known as the vice principal. She had a stumpy build like an egg-shaped Weeble, black scraggly hair, and warts all over her face. Okay, maybe they were moles—but not sexy moles like Cindy Crawford, more like troll-living-under-a-bridge moles.

Imagine Principal Barbie and the Wicked Witch of the West in a Disney movie where the princess was beautiful and the evil antagonist was frightening. They were kinda like that.

Then there was my team, which consisted of the other four second grade teachers—each one of them oozing with confidence and likability. All four of them were beautiful—perfect boobs, perfect nails, perfect hair, perfect clothes. They had matching T-shirts for every occasion.

Welcome to Second Grade—matching T-shirts.

Election Day—matching T-shirts.

Earth Day—matching T-shirts.

National Rubber Ducky Day—matching T-shirts.

All four of them decorated their classrooms without silly fire codes getting in the way. They burnt a wickless candle each day, hung 10,000 art projects from the ceiling, put decorative baskets and other froufrou items on top of their cabinets, and draped the walls with twinkling lights. These were all big no-no's at my Chicago school, but I didn't want to be outdone, so I joined in. A few weeks into the school year, we all had to take everything down for the fire department's scheduled visit. Then we put it all back up the following day. Principal Barbie knew we did that, but she was a strong supporter of the greater good—a school fit for a Barbie.

I thought that second grade team would be my people. Every best friend in my life—Rachel, Ben, Anna, and Molly—had all fallen in the "beautiful, popular, confident, over-achiever" category. I felt like the second grade team was made especially for me, but I was so wrong.

Finally, there was Aidan. Adorable, little, pain-in-my-ass Aidan. This was my eighteenth year of teaching, so I'd taught every type of student, especially coming from an all-inclusive school. One year, I had a student whose behavior was described to me as "like a caged animal." That student became one of my all-time favorites. He gave me such big hugs that he'd lift me off the ground. The "naughty" kids have always held a special place in my heart—maybe because I was naughty; maybe because I loved making a positive impact in their lives; maybe because I hoped Greyson's teachers treated him the same way. I'm not exactly sure of the reason, but I always connected with the troublemakers.

But that year my job shifted from second grade teacher to security guard.

Aidan would forcefully snip scissors at his classmates' faces. He'd peel the metal part off a pencil, break it into tiny bits, then flick the pieces at students' faces. He'd crumble the little eraser on top of the pencil, put the pieces in his mouth, then spit them at students. Aidan would go from student to student poking them with staples, paper clips, sharpened pencils, and tacks. He'd push his thumbs into students' eyes, pull their hair, and scream in their ears. He'd laugh out loud when kids got answers wrong. He'd drum on his desk with pencils, glue sticks, anything he could get his hands on. When I tried to take items away from him, he'd hold onto them with all his might. He would sing, hum, oink, bark, and howl during instruction and tests. If I asked him to stop, he'd do it louder. He'd crawl on the floor, climb on the desks, and flip his chair. He'd dump the large bucket that held the students' lunches, crawl in, and roll around the room. He'd pretend to shoot students with pencils, glue bottles—anything that resembled a gun. He'd use the same items up against students' necks, pretending he had a knife. He'd steal things from me, color on the carpet, and destroy my personal materials and classroom supplies. When I tried to manage his behavior, he'd throw tantrums like a toddler or chest-bump me and say, "You ain't the boss of me." He'd leave my classroom and roam the school without permission, throw chairs down the hallway, and barricade the door so no one could get out.

I tried every trick up my sleeve with Aidan: positive behavior charts with stickers, special classroom jobs, insane amounts of praise. If Aidan did so much as sit at his desk for five minutes, I enthusiastically said, "I love how nicely you're sitting." Students normally eat that stuff up, but no, not Aidan.

Aidan's mom never sent a snack, so I bought all his favorite snacks and gave him one each day. I tutored him every day after school because he was so far behind academically. Aidan cherished his time with me after school; he was a different boy in a one-on-one setting. With any other student in the universe, that type of attention would drastically reduce behavior problems in the classroom. But no, not Aidan.

In Aidan's defense, if he were at my school in suburban Chicago, he would've received a one-on-one teaching assistant to take him on breaks throughout the day, redirect negative behaviors, and offer academic support. He would've been tutored every day by a reading specialist and weekly by a math interventionist, occupational therapist, and school psychologist. But at Shitsville Elementary, there were no interventions. Everything fell on the classroom teacher. *Toto, I don't think we're in Chicago anymore.*

I scheduled a meeting with Principal Barbie and explained Aidan's behavior. I showed her all my notes on Aidan. I told her it was just a matter of time before he hurt someone. Principal Barbie told me to write a referral to send Aidan to the office every time he endangered a student. I had never written a referral in my life, but Principal Barbie seemed so enthusiastic to help with her unwavering smile, cheerful voice, and flowery designer dress, so I agreed.

I was only a month into my job and when I wasn't working, I was begging Greyson to move to Florida. My cousin lived in Florida, and she was a doctor—an excellent, highly respected, award-winning doctor. Dr. Doctor's whole life revolved around one thing: being a doctor. She was married to her job, leaving her no time for men, friends, or fun. Just work, work, work, work, work. *She makes my teeny tiny list of great doctors.*

Dr. Doctor agreed to try to help Greyson. She bravely invited him to live with her, even though I'd told her everything. I told her to lock her bedroom door at night. She was, quite literally, my very last hope.

Shockingly, Greyson agreed to move in with Dr. Doctor.

Dr. Doctor wasn't home often, but when she was, she took firsthand notes on Greyson. We spoke regularly, and I listened to her skirt around her thoughts about him, like she was still trying to figure Greyson out. Or maybe he was standing behind her with an ax . . . not sure.

Dr. Doctor told me about Greyson's frightening behaviors, like how he spent his days locked in his bedroom. When she'd try to talk to him, *if* he answered, it was through the closed door. When she'd insist that he open the door, he'd open it an inch and talk through the crack, glaring at her with one of his white eyes. She'd try to interact with him when he went to the kitchen. She certainly never caught him on his way to use the shower or restroom.

None of Dr. Doctor's reports about Greyson surprised me. Until one day when I was pressuring her to give me her diagnosis.

"Dr. Doctor, gimme the news." *All right, maybe I didn't say that.* "Does Greyson really have schizophrenia or schizoaffective disorder?"

"Worse."

"Worse?! What the hell could be worse?!"

"Personality disorder."

Personality disorder is a mental disorder that causes an inflexible and unhealthy pattern of thinking, functioning, and behaving. There are several types of personality disorder, and Greyson displays characteristics from almost all of them. Personality disorder causes Greyson to prefer solitary activities and isolation. He has a restricted range of emotions and an unawareness of other people's feelings, so he shows little to no remorse about the effects of his behavior. When communicating with Greyson, his beliefs manifest in unusual speech that either consists of circular, overelaborate monologues or extremely minimal (or nonexistent) verbal exchanges with misplaced long silences, during which he says one word, gazes off in the distance for a few minutes, and then says the next word. During conversations, he reacts either inappropriately or not at all. He displays odd behaviors, paranoid fears, suspiciousness, and a grandiose sense of self-importance. He displays a sense of entitlement, believing he is exceptionally unique and can only be understood by an elite few. Greyson views the world in extremes—all is good or all is bad—and his opinions change quickly. He has recurring thoughts of suicidal behaviors and hears voices that tell him he should die. He has difficulty trusting and an irrational fear of other people's intentions. He is secretive, emotionally cold, and excessively serious. Greyson also has strange beliefs and magical thinking—like being convinced that glass jars and organic futons have magical powers.

Personality disorder (particularly cluster A, which includes schizotypal, schizoid, and paranoid personality disorders) at its core is very similar to schizophrenia, and schizophrenia falls under the schizoaffective disorder umbrella. All three mental health disorders are related and have overlapping characteristics. So does Greyson have all three? Depends which doctor you ask.

It's okay. I'm confused too.

Dr. Doctor did gimme some good news, though. I'm not sure how she did it, but she managed to get Greyson into a government office to sign the required paperwork to receive money, food stamps, and medical care. Then, after hours on the phone and all day at the social security office, I became Greyson's representative payee so I could control his finances. Unfortunately, government assistance only lasted two years. To clarify, to continue assistance, I'd have to endure the whole hellacious process all over again every two years. Apparently, the government thinks a person with Greyson's diagnoses can possibly work full-time. Perhaps he could get a job where plastic bags are readily available for him to shit in, like a fast-food joint.

I was temporarily less burdened financially, but emotionally, Greyson's latest diagnosis made me ill. I couldn't believe the boy I loved so wholeheartedly was diagnosed with the same mental disorder as Charles Manson, who, by the way, was admittedly Greyson's idol. Greyson found him "fascinating and brilliant."

After Dr. Doctor let Greyson live with her for a month, he moved on to his next apartment. I will be forever grateful that Dr. Doctor took Greyson in, studied him, and got him on government assistance. However, Dr. Doctor also voiced her opinion that I was a bad mom for kicking Greyson out of the house. That crushed me. Dr. Doctor and I had always lived in different states, and we've gone as long as a decade without seeing one another. I think she's met Greyson twice. She had absolutely no idea what kind of mom I was or how I'd fought for Greyson the first twenty-one years of his life. She had no idea how much abuse I'd endured or the impact

Greyson had had on my health, my marriage, my life. And she expected me to raise my two young children under the same roof as Greyson, surrounded by that same abuse. *There really should be a law about people without children giving parenting advice.*

Dr. Doctor thought, at the very least, I should fly out regularly to see Greyson. That made sense . . . on the surface. And I did visit Greyson—once. I took him out to dinner and he just stared off in the distance. All my questions received one-word answers or no acknowledgment at all. I took him to Target to shop. He threw things in my cart, but didn't humor me with interaction.

Maybe I am *awful. Maybe I should throw airfare and hotel stays (in exchange for interactionless visits) on my Greyson expenditures list.* I guess I was no longer willing to rearrange my life around Greyson, no longer willing to put myself in a situation where I didn't feel safe, no longer willing to take precious time away from Violet and Rockwell. I gave Greyson all of me for so long, and I just couldn't anymore. I was tapped out. Since I'd found out I was pregnant with Greyson, I hadn't lived my life—even a little bit—for me.

A TEACHER, A BARBIE, AND A WITCH WALK INTO A BAR

2015–2016

*M*y year at Shitsville Elementary wasn't the Claire year I had hoped for. I did exactly as I was told by Principal Barbie. I wrote a detailed referral every single day for weeks since Aidan endangered my students multiple times a day. But nothing ever happened. It was like the referrals just . . . disappeared.

Even the referral I wrote after a field trip to a theater downtown just seemed to vanish into thin air. A student of mine, Melody, was on her tippy toes looking over a bridge with a thirty-foot drop. Aidan came up from behind her, held her tight around her ankles, and stood up quickly, lifting her over the edge of the bridge. Thankfully, when I screamed, he stopped.

I told Principal Barbie what happened as soon as we returned from the field trip, and she saw the fear in my eyes. I wrote the referral and asked Principal Barbie to call Melody's mother. I felt it was more appropriate for the principal to handle such a severe incident. But nothing was done. I later found out no phone call was ever made. The incident was completely ignored.

Why did Principal Barbie tell me to write referrals if she was just going to ignore them?

Suddenly, it became clear when the Wicked Witch of the West pulled me aside after a staff meeting. She looked at me, square in the eyes, with a you-don't-know-who-you're-fucking-with look, and sternly said, "You know . . . I really like Aidan. I mean, I really, REALLY like Aidan."

That was all she said.

Hey Freak Show, I like Aidan, too, so maybe we should work together to help him.

For Lord knows why, the Wicked Witch of the West threatened me and basically ordered me to leave Aidan alone. She had some sort of twisted agenda, and I knew in that moment my career at Shitsville Elementary was over before it began. When I told the second grade team what had happened, they didn't believe me.

After the Wicked Witch of the West threatened me less than two months into the school year, Principal Barbie never spoke to me again. Never—not one single word. I stopped writing referrals. I just did my job and prayed to God that Aidan wouldn't hurt anyone.

However, I did continue to take detailed notes on Aidan's behavior. A coworker who'd witnessed his behavior asked me why I wasn't writing referrals. She didn't believe me when I told her the story. She asked if she could show Principal Barbie all my notes. *Be my guest. Maybe now Principal Barbie will sit down with me so we can come up with a plan to help Aidan. Ha, just kidding!* I still never heard one word from Principal Barbie.

The Wicked Witch of the West enjoyed taunting me throughout the school year. She often popped into my classroom, thumbed through the personal belongings on my desk, and glared at me as I taught. She left notes stating things like, "You should've pulled your low students for academic support during that art project." In other words, she wanted me to single out my academically low students and punish them by not allowing them to do art. *Great suggestion, moron!*

The Wicked Witch of the West loved getting under my skin because she knew I'd just bend over and take it, just like I did with my second grade team. No, I never made friends that year. Not at Shitsville Elementary where the second grade team was just like me—Chicago me. They were very social, very cheery, very teacher-y, very cliquey. Five years earlier, I would've swooped in and shined like Kate Middleton entering the royal family. But instead, their four classrooms made a square in the hallway and then there was me, way off to the side. Even geographically, I was an outsider. They would hang out in their square, laughing and giggling like I used to do at my school in Chicago. It was a laugh that said, "Look how much people love me! Look how good I look! Ha, ha, ha! Good Lord, I'm so funny!"

Then for our district-wide meetings, they carpooled without me. (After all, a Mercedes only seats four.) They walked in the door, Starbucks in hand, flipping their beautiful hair, wearing their designer clothes, and laughing their telling laughs. Waving their strong bond in my face every day slowly crushed my spirit.

I started to regret leaving Chicago, my amazing job, and all my friends behind. I was going through culture shock because—spoiler alert—California was nothing like Chicago. After so many years, I had forgotten how different it was. I felt like I'd moved to an alternate universe. *People don't even know what an Italian beef is here, and they think Domino's is a good pizza. It's downright criminal!*

Every ounce of happiness I could muster at work was saved for my students. At least *they* loved me—they all lit up and ran to hug me when they arrived at school each day.

Even Aidan flashed his toothy grin and gave me a huge hug. He was slowly getting better, albeit at a molasses-like speed.

But around the second grade team, I was not in the mood for hair flips and giggles. I wanted to grab them and say, *Listen, I'm usually a barrel of fucking laughs, but my son was recently diagnosed with schizophrenia, schizoaffective disorder, and personality disorder. And you wouldn't even believe the last five years I've had. Oh, and I just moved across the country, leaving my wonderful job, a comfortable home, and all my friends behind— only to get replaced with an awful job, a crap apartment, and you four bitches.*

I especially wanted to do that near the end of the school year when one of the teachers was in tears—literally full-on tears—because she was so stressed over having a new in-ground pool installed.

(Insert slobbery, squeaky voice here.) "I didn't realize how stressful getting a pool was."

Tear, tear.

Cry, cry.

Sad, sad.

Ya wanna know what stressful is beotch? I'll tell you what stressful is. Stressful is having a son who's been moving from apartment to house to apartment to house—living in mental health hospitals or on the streets in between each move. All. School. Year. Long.

With every move, I had grueling exchanges with Greyson about where he should go and what he should do. With every move, I searched for a new place for him, even though I knew he wouldn't listen. With every move, I had conversations with landlords forewarning them that Greyson had some serious issues. (I quickly learned that rent coming from a reliable source took precedence over my carefully voiced concerns.) With every move, I continued to pay another first and last months' rent plus security deposit,

292 | THE SAD SON

which—news flash—I never got back. With every move, I continued to buy Greyson all new belongings since he always left everything behind.

During that year, Greyson lived with roommates until they slowly picked up on his unorthodox behavior. Greyson came out of his room for only one reason—to get food. When he did come out of his room, he filled the kitchen with his repugnant smell. He'd fill a filthy, never-washed glass jar with his raw, unpasteurized milk. Then he'd top a filthy, never-washed plate with rotten food, and he never used utensils to eat. He'd sometimes consume things like an entire bag of Himalayan salt or a whole bottle of coconut oil. It wouldn't take long for Greyson's roommates to notice that he never used the bathroom—not to shower, not to brush his teeth, not to wash his hands, not to use the toilet. They noticed Greyson only wore one outfit—one outfit that was never washed. They started to hear him laughing, talking, and screaming as though he wasn't alone in his room, saying things like, "When everyone around me is drowning, I float"—over and over and over. They heard Greyson make proclamations like, "I hereby institute the Church of Futon— the Protector of Everything."

Eventually, Greyson's roommates made the connection that cockroaches had moved in at the same time as him. Eventually, his roommates became curious. Eventually, his roommates decided to take a peek in Greyson's room when he left for the grocery store.

When they peeked into Greyson's room, they saw the cockroaches scatter. They saw the window, the mirror, and the TV screen covered with black, plastic bags. When they peeked into Greyson's room, they smelled urine, bowel movements, and rotten food. They saw a floor covered with half-eaten fruit, old potato peels, and glass jars full of piss. When they peeked into Greyson's room, they saw his brand-new organic futon soiled with sauces, mysterious liquids, scraps of food, and duct tape. When they lifted the corner of the futon, they saw mold growing underneath. When they peeked into Greyson's room, they saw a sixty-gallon container overflowing with trash—some of it unidentifiable.

Eventually, his roommates became scared. I know this because they sent me e-mails. I know this because they sent me pictures. I know this because I lived it.

Some roommates called an exterminator. This led to Greyson screaming—for hours—that they were poisoning him.

Some roommates called the police. Each time, the police sent Greyson to a mental health hospital. Just like in Chicago, he was out after one to three days.

Some roommates called the health department. This led to the disposal of Greyson's brand-new organic futon. Yes, I purchased a new $900 organic futon every time he moved. He believed organic futons had "magical powers," so he *needed* an organic futon to survive. He relentlessly harassed me and screamed at me until I caved.

Even though Greyson received government assistance, I was spending hundreds, sometimes thousands, of dollars each month.

Now that, my dear, is stress. Choosing the perfect tile for your new in-ground pool is not.

My year at Shitsville Elementary did, however, end with some superfun information. A different teacher at my school suggested that I call the president of the teacher's association when she caught me crying after the Wicked Witch of the West had had her way with me again. So I called him, just for kicks, and told him about my experience. Turns out that the Wicked Witch of the West formerly held a director position at the district office, but she'd been demoted to vice principal. Apparently, she'd had multiple grievances filed against her by several teachers in the district. I also found out . . . wait for it . . . a group of teachers filed a lawsuit against her, and *WON*! Furthermore, (I told you these were fun!) I learned that Principal Barbie had married a wealthy man over twice her age and had "submitted her resignation" at the end of the year, which I'm putting in quotes because the president told me she may have been asked to resign. And, this may be my favorite part, but I can't decide because I love them all, when the Wicked Witch of the West applied to fill Principal Barbie's position, she got a big fat *NO*. They can't fire her, but they can make her vice principal . . . forever.

Can you believe I worked for these clowns?

When my one-year temporary contract at the school expired, neither I nor the principals asked for an extension. When parents found out I was leaving, they were very upset. Two of them showed me e-mails they'd written to the superintendent praising me. But no one, absolutely no one, was more upset than Aidan. Yes, Aidan, the boy who triggered the fuck-filled avalanche I endured all year. He found out I was leaving at the end of the last day of school. I'll never forget that moment. He cried and he cried, and he held me tight, then he slowly shuffled toward the door, his head drooping, tears dripping off his nose. Then he stopped, turned around, and our teary eyes locked for moment, marking my very last day at Shitsville Elementary.

THE SAD ME

2016

*M*y parents went on a cruise—a thirty-five-day European cruise. Good for them, I know, but terrible for me. My life was a mess, and I wouldn't be able to talk to them for a month. *Yeah, yeah, I realize how bratty I sound. What's your point?* I would've been happier for them if they hadn't already taken, like, fifty other cruises since retiring.

I applied for teaching jobs. Again. (Long, drawn-out sigh.) Under normal circumstances, I'd be excited to get offered multiple teaching positions. But, as the offers rolled in, my heart felt heavy, my stomach felt sick. Something—maybe everything—wasn't right.

Then I was called to interview for a part-time teaching position at a nearby district where I'd just interviewed for a full-time position. The part-time position was at the district's alternative school. Well, of course I said, "No, thank you." I mean, part-time, alternative school—sounds awful. I can see it now—making half a paycheck, teaching in a school full of little Aidans with zero support (since I was still in California). No, thank you.

But I kept thinking about that interview for whatever reason. A couple days went by and there I was, still thinking about that interview. I gave the district a call back and asked if they were still scheduling interviews for that position. They said yes, and I interviewed the next day.

I ended up getting offered both positions—the part-time and the full-time. The lady in the office laughed when she called to give me the news—like I'd cheated somehow. All my interviews with other districts were fluff. This was the district I wanted, but they rarely had openings. In fact, those were the only two open elementary teacher positions that year. The year before, they didn't have any.

I was annoyed with myself that I was considering the part-time position. If I could've talked to my dad, I knew exactly what he'd say. "Take the full-time position, Claire. You and Michael just bought a new house. You can't afford that home on half a salary. Plus, think about your retirement. You've got to work toward your retirement, Claire."

Yes, I could hear my logical father as clear as day, even though he was somewhere in the middle of the ocean. But he didn't really say that because he had no idea I was offered both positions. So, technically, I wouldn't be ignoring my dad's advice if I took the part-time job. Not that I do everything my dad says. If I did, I would've never dated Sperm Donor, been a single mom, or left my wonderful job in Chicago. So take that, Dad.

Michael and I discussed my options at great length, but we wished my dad could weigh in. Not to get his opinion, since we already knew it. We wanted my dad to persuade me into making the sensible decision because we were both leaning toward the insensible, go-into-debt decision.

"Hi, Mrs. Smith! It's Claire Josephine. I'd like to accept the part-time teaching position at the alternative school."

"Um. . . . Are you sure?"

"Yes." *No.* "I'm sure." *Sure that I'm crazy.*

My new teaching job was a cakewalk. And I mean that in the best possible way. It was so easy—no classroom management, no decorating a classroom, no endless hours of grading, no formal parent conferences, no formal observations, no endless hours of planning lessons. In other words, no stress. I basically worked one-on-one with students who couldn't attend a traditional school. Some students were athletes, some were actors, some had mental health issues, some had behavioral issues. Students came in and out of the program, but I averaged only around ten students at a time. *TEN!* If they were in third grade or above, they used an online curriculum. If they were in first or second grade, I created the curriculum. I even made my own schedule. Can you believe it? My own schedule! My principal told me not to work more than seventeen and a half hours a week, per my contract. Can you imagine? I was being told to watch my hours! I went from working my ass off to working seventeen and a half hours per week. Seventeen and a half! Ha! It's comical how few hours I worked. Yes, my paycheck was cut in half, but it felt like a win because my hours were cut by about 70 percent. It was just what the doctor ordered after a year at Shitsville. Yes, we had to sell some of Michael's company stock options just to survive, *BUT*, my family was being vastly rewarded with home-cooked meals, plus our kids got their mom back, and Michael had a wife who was no longer sobbing daily over a job she despised.

At least my work tears were eliminated. During my year at Shitsville, my work tears usually occurred on my drive home, which resulted in me walking through the door a blubbering mess. Other times my work tears emerged when I'd call Michael at lunch to tell him how my cliquey team made me feel like an outcast. Again. Those were my prime-time tears. Michael got stuck with those tears.

But my Greyson tears . . . those tears will never be eliminated. Luckily for Michael, he's generally off the hook for the Greyson tears. Those tears predominantly happen late at night.

At night, after the kids and Michael go to bed, I usually watch some TV. Maybe it's to relax, maybe it's to torture myself, I'm not sure. Sometimes I think TV and movies are my nemesis.

It seems as though everything I watch reminds me of Greyson. Every time I watch a mom giving birth on TV, I cry. I reminisce about the day Greyson was born and what it felt like to hold him for the first time. His eyes were so bright. His little nose was so cute. He had all his fingers and toes. He was so beautiful, so innocent, so sweet. He didn't even cry. I think about how, in that perfect moment, I was bursting with love, hope, and joy. That flicker in time felt so flawless. I was young, naive, and unsuspecting that a perfect little being could be mentally ill—that my bundle of joy was actually a bundle of sadness. I wish I could've bottled that first precious moment with Greyson so that now when I see a newborn on TV, on Facebook, or in a stroller passing by, I could open it up and feel that moment again, instead of feeling so much pain.

Then there are those moments on TV when someone reaches a milestone—big or small, doesn't matter. Someone gets their driver's license, makes a friend, goes off to college, graduates, lands a job, earns a promotion, wins a girl's heart, gets married, buys their first home. All the things you see on TV every day. When most people see simple milestones on TV, they just watch their show and eat their chips. But for me, watching those milestones are nightly reminders of what Greyson will never do. They remind me of things I'll never get to watch him experience—all the good things in life he's never going to have. I find myself crying during scenes that most find mundane. Even watching simple exchanges between a mother and son make me cry.

I want to visit Greyson in his dorm. I want to meet his college buddies. I want to embarrass him in front of his girlfriend. I want to be there when he has his first heartbreak. I want to support him when he chooses an occupation. I want to cheer him up when he doesn't land a job. I want to celebrate with him when he does. I want to watch Greyson's face as his bride walks down the aisle. I want to buy him a toaster and bath towels when he buys his first home. I want to love and hold his children. But Greyson and I will never have those moments—neither the special, nor the mundane.

But the hardest shows to watch are the reality shows. Seeing a proud parent in the audience gets me every time. I tear up when the camera captures a mother's face full of joy or those segments when they film a mom talking about her son with such pride, saying things like, "I knew my son was special ever since he was a little boy." I want to scream at the TV that I knew my son was special too. But I'll never have that again—that feeling of being proud of Greyson. I'll never have that look of pride the camera always seems to capture and throw in my face.

My other nemeses are the holidays. Every holiday is brutal, but Halloween and Christmas are the worst. I tried so hard to make holiday traditions for Greyson that I now try so hard to forget. Every Halloween, I'm reminded of all the fun things we did. All the hayrides we went on, the pumpkin patches we frequented, the haunted houses we made for Greyson's annual Halloween party. I sold all our decorations before we moved. As people walked away toting our skeletons and zombies, I had flashes of how excited Greyson and I were when we scored them for half price after Halloween. Selling everything was supposed to make the pain go away. But it didn't. Instead, I'm just left with a humdrum house on Halloween—the kind of house Greyson and I used to pity.

Halloween is bad, but Christmas is worse. I torment myself with daydreams of Greyson walking through the door, balancing an armful of poorly wrapped Christmas presents for his little brother and sister. Then Violet and Rockwell run down the stairs yelling, "Greyson's here! Greyson's here!" They giggle and hang on his legs with all their might while he walks and makes monster sounds. Then Greyson makes a silly comment about how Santa doesn't visit kids who giggle as he sets down the presents and tickles Violet and Rockwell on the floor. I picture Violet and Rockwell proudly presenting Greyson with their handmade gifts, and he pretends they're the greatest gifts in the world. I can see Greyson and I fighting over the stuffing at Christmas dinner then watching cheesy Christmas movies all night. And I can actually laugh instead of cry when I watch them. That's what Christmas is supposed to look like. But it will never look like that. I'll always have a hole in my heart at Christmas.

Then I have my prayer cries. For the first fifteen years of Greyson's life, I thanked God every night for blessing me with an extraordinary genius. I would have conversations with God telling him how I couldn't wait to see what kind of man Greyson would become. I always felt like God had chosen me—like I was the chosen one to raise the mastermind. Then, when Greyson was sixteen, my prayers shifted. I started praying every night that Greyson would get better. *Please Lord, let this be a phase.* After that, I stopped knowing how to pray for Greyson. After years of praying for Greyson to get better, he only got worse. I started praying to God to just "do whatever" is in His plan for Greyson, as if I ever had a say. *You do have a plan, right, God?* I don't understand why He would put a boy on this earth just to be sad, just to break my heart.

I've even found myself praying to God to just take Greyson. *Just take him. Please.* I just want Greyson's suffering to be over. Let him be with You in heaven where he'll no longer be mentally ill. Greyson tells me he hears voices that tell him to kill himself, that he feels like a lifeless corpse, that he's always in pain—in pain from his rotted teeth and his frail body. I often wonder who will find Greyson dead. It's ironic that for so many years I prayed for God to watch over him, *Please Lord, keep Greyson healthy and safe.* Now I pray for the excruciating pain he calls life to just be over.

I wonder sometimes if I deserve Greyson—that maybe this is karma at its finest. Most people didn't like me when I was young for a reason—or several—but I've grown, significantly. I'm unrecognizable to my high school self. I don't know, but sometimes I wonder if God is punishing me for all my mistakes. I may not be perfect or have all the answers like born-again Christians think they do, but I'm pretty sure God doesn't function that way. I'm pretty sure God is sad that I'm sad because Greyson is sad.

I think about how much I sacrificed for Greyson. I was so careful during my pregnancy, stayed home with him the first few years, didn't date for seven years in my twenties, gave up material things, and completely revolved every aspect of my life around him. I think about every birthday and Halloween party I hosted, every annual pass we had to frequent all the fun places, every picnic I packed for our long days at the park. All the board games we played, all the books I read, all the puzzles we did. All the stupid hills I sled down in freezing cold temperatures, all the crappy Chuck E. Cheese pizza I ate, and all the Pokémon movies I suffered through. I did all that not only because I loved Greyson with all my heart, but because I looked at every single thing I did as an investment in his future.

I invested in Greyson's future with every note I put in his beautifully made lunches and by never missing a single opportunity to tuck him in at night. I invested in Greyson's future by never having much yet making sure he was never in need of anything. I invested in Greyson's future by providing ongoing, memorable, Greyson-centered life experiences, but to this day, I have only had one adult vacation in my life.

I taught Greyson all the things a good mom should teach:

- money management with an allowance and trips to the bank
- responsibility by giving him chores
- gratitude by volunteering at a food bank
- sportsmanship through organized sports
- family values through countless holiday traditions
- morals by not allowing men in and out of his life
- strength by showing him everything a single mom can do
- pride by prevailing without the help of Sperm Donor
- tenacity through education to earn a master's degree
- a strong work ethic by example
- love by mine never wavering
- faith through prayer and years of attending church
- devotion by giving him all of me for two decades

And what was it all for? Nothing. Absolutely nothing. Not a damn thing! He's none of those things. It kills me that my very best efforts spanning over twenty years were rewarded with literally nothing—like my life has been one big practical joke. All the classes I've taken, all the workshops I've attended, all the seminars I've sat through, and all the books I've read that said, "If you do this, this, this, and this, you'll raise a happy and successful child." *Ha, ha, ha! Just kidding Claire. Joke's on you.*

But the worst part, by far, the part that makes me feel sick, is how Greyson has suffered. I would endure what I've been through a million times over if it would help him. I would die to give Greyson a healthy brain. It crushes me to think how this sweet little baby never stood a chance in the world. He's gone through life trapped in a body with an incurable mind. How torturous it must be. How helpless he must feel. The thought gives me indescribable pain. Why Greyson? He doesn't deserve this. Why does Greyson have to suffer because I had sex with an awful man?

Greyson's life is all my fault. I caused this. Greyson has suffered because of ME.

Many people believe things happen for a reason. Good God, I hope that's true. If it is, then I had a shit algebra teacher *for a reason*. I failed her class, couldn't try out for cheer or dance, and left my high school senior year to meet Sperm Donor *for a reason*. I then visited my parents, made plans with a friend, and ran into Sperm Donor that night *for a reason*. I was fooled, fell in love, and had unprotected sex, once, *for a reason*. The mentally ill sperm made its way to the egg during an "impossible time to get pregnant" *for a reason*. I revolved my entire life around an unhealthy brain and tormented soul for two solid decades *for a reason*. Then I left Chicago and my wonderful job for the worst job with the worst boss with the worst student in the worst district in the worst state *for a reason*.

Maybe God knew that was the only way I'd take a break from teaching. Maybe God knew my father had to be on that cruise ship when I was deciding between a full-time and part-time job. Maybe God was that voice that told me to take the part-time job so I could write this book.

A book I hope helps other moms of children with disabilities to not feel so alone. A book to possibly shed some light on the laws regarding financial and psychiatric assistance. A book to encourage others not to be so judgmental of the mentally ill and the parents who raise them. A book that maybe persuades you to embrace someone who could really use a friend. A book advising young adults to think before having sex or getting into someone's car. A book asking born-again Christians to practice what they preach. A book that proves your instincts are your superpower. A book to hopefully make you think, but also laugh a little. A book that is my last-ditch effort to get the resources I need to help a son I love get stable housing and care that I can't afford.

A book about my son.

The sad son.

"*M*y whole life, never once did I feel like you didn't love me," Greyson said to me out of the blue during our last conversation. I had to mute the phone so I could bawl happy tears while he continued to reminisce over some childhood memories. Then Greyson's girlfriend chimed in (they were both talking to me on speakerphone), saying she doesn't have any happy memories of her mom. Greyson's response to her was, "Well, my mom is an exception to the rule. We did *everything* together."

I cried for a good hour after that call.

A lot has changed in the three years it took me to write this book—well, one year to write it and two years to revise and edit it. Revising and editing took longer because I went back to teaching full-time and also developed some worsening health issues. (Remember that epidural I had in 2010 when Rockwell was born? Yep, I still suffer from central nervous system issues.) I also went through a divorce, taking all Michaels in the universe—unless his last name is Jordan—officially off the table *forEVER*.

But your primary interest is probably not my job, my

health, or my love life—except you dirty scoundrels who read the chapter on Sam and our sex life twice. (PS—You're my favorite readers.) That said, Greyson's transformation from what I'd describe as "on the verge of death" to having a coherent and—on this particular day—lovely conversation with me did not happen overnight. In the fall of 2016—around the time I started writing this book—Greyson called me and said he was temporarily homeless after getting kicked out of yet another house and being released from another mental health hospital. He was twenty-two years old and was about to move into an apartment, which would double the cost of his rent because he had been renting a single room in a house. I had mixed feelings about Greyson living in an apartment alone. On the one hand, there would be no one to send me pictures or updates. But on the upside, it would take longer for him to get kicked out because his unusual behaviors would take a lot longer to detect. And taking longer to get kicked out equaled more time before I'd lose another security deposit and last month's rent. Still, I really wanted roommates keeping an eye on him, yet I felt so bad about putting other people in that position. It really was a lose-lose situation.

"Greyson, why do you need your own apartment? The rent on that place will eat up your entire monthly financial assistance," I said exasperated—again—knowing whatever I said wouldn't matter and that I'd continue supporting him financially until the end of time.

"My girlfriend is moving in with me, so she'll pay half the rent," he responded nonchalantly, as if what he'd just said made complete sense.

I took a deep breath, made the sign of the cross, and said between clenched teeth, "Your *girlfriend*? What *girlfriend*?"

"Eva. She's just waiting to turn eighteen so she can move in with me."

Insert heart attack here.

"Eva—a girl who I've never once heard you mention—is moving in with you when she turns (trying to keep it cool but losing it here) *EIGHTEEN*?" I growled while internally contemplating giving Eva some credit for waiting to move in until she was legal.

"Yep."

"So where'd ya meet?" I said, trying to sound casual. *On the street? In a mental health hospital? Maybe she's a hallucination.*

"Online."

Perfect. Totally fuckin' perfect, I thought. "Have you two *even* met . . . like in person?" I attempted to ask without skepticism in my voice but failed miserably.

"No."

"How did you meet online?" *I'm fascinated, tell me more.*

"She discovered my blog."

"Does she know you just got kicked out of a house and released from a mental health hospital (again)?" *And more importantly, does her mother know?*

"Yep."

"Don't you think she's a bit young?"

"You and dad are four years apart." *I was hoping you wouldn't remember that.*

"When do you expect her to move in?" Trying to act like I totally thought it would actually happen.

"In a few weeks."

"Okay, talk soon."

That was an interesting turn of events I definitely wasn't expecting. *You've really outdone yourself this time God.*

After I told Michael the news, we proceeded to place bets on how long their courtship would last. Michael bet on a week. I bet on an entire month, knowing that an eighteen-year-old girl who was drawn to Greyson's obscure, unorthodox, intermittent blog, which documented his extreme views, couldn't be too intuitive. Then we anxiously waited to see if Eva was an actual live human.

Sure enough, a few weeks later, she moved in.

Eva and I spoke on the phone, and I quickly learned what kind of eighteen-year-old girl moves in—voluntarily—with a twenty-two-year-old man she discovered online.

Eva had spent her earliest years living in a poor country. Eva's father abandoned her as a baby, and her mother was mentally and physically abusive, so her schizophrenic grandmother primarily raised her. After moving to the United States, Eva attended military school at her mother's insistence. As a result, Eva had to spend four hours a day on public transportation getting to and from school.

All her life, Eva has suffered from severe mental and physical health conditions (plus an additional one every time we speak), which qualifies her for government assistance. She is, however, very intelligent in a Greyson-sorta way.

Their first year together was simply a continuation of Greyson's previous experiences with roommates: they fought nonstop, Eva kept calling the police, and Greyson was in and out of mental health hospitals. You know how most people end phone calls with "I love you"? I ended our phone calls with "Don't get pregnant!"

I felt overwhelming guilt that an eighteen-year-old girl was caring for Greyson, so I spent the first year trying to save Eva. "You know, Eva, you don't *have* to be with Greyson. You're young and have your whole life ahead of you. You're a smart, beautiful girl and deserve to be treated well," I continuously said to her during that first year.

"Living with Greyson is better than living with my mom," she'd respond.

"Living with Greyson or your mom aren't your only options," I'd point out, but my advice fell on deaf ears. I have that effect on teenagers.

But gradually, something unforeseen happened: Eva convinced Greyson to see doctors. Then slowly, something unbelievable happened: Eva convinced Greyson to see psychologists. And finally, something phenomenal happened: Eva convinced Greyson to take medicine.

And the unanticipated perk—which could only come from living with an intelligent hypochondriac who was abused by her mother and raised by her schizophrenic grandma—was that Eva had loads of knowledge about schizophrenia and prescriptions. Plus, she had an extreme tolerance for . . . well, anything insufferable.

Eva worked closely with Greyson's doctors to get the right combination of medicines. She researched every new prescription and documented every side effect he experienced. She logged all of Greyson's mood and behavioral changes and argued with doctors who didn't have Greyson's best interests in mind. In other words, Greyson managed to find the one person in the entire universe —*literally*—who could handle him. If it weren't for Eva, Greyson would likely be dead.

Fast-forward to the beginning of 2020. As I prepare to publish my memoir, Eva and Greyson are still together, legitimately proving that even when I'm 100 percent, unequivocally certain of something, I can still manage to be wrong.

Over the years, Eva and I have formed a close relationship. I talk to her and Greyson on the phone weekly. The two of them wear wedding rings, but they're not legally married. Still, I consider her my daughter-in-law, and, more than anything, I want to take care of her and Greyson. I feel extreme gratitude for all Eva has done for Greyson.

Thanks to Eva, Greyson is doing well . . . for a man with his diagnoses. Eva still complains about his pee jars (*and rightly so*), the cockroaches and maggots he attracts into their apartment (*I can't argue with her on that*), and his magical beliefs that his mattress has powers (*now she's just being nitpicky*). He still hears voices, but they've stopped telling him to die and are much more manageable. He also lives a completely sedentary life, meaning that he lays on his magical mattress with as little movement as possible (hence the pee jars and mini fridge within reach of his mattress) for nearly twenty-four hours a day—sleeping for about twelve of them. Greyson only leaves the apartment (or moves for that matter) to go to the grocery store once or twice a month or to go to his doctor's appointments. Greyson's sedentary life works for Eva because it's difficult for her to be mobile with all her medical conditions, which I won't attempt to list or pretend that I understand.

Greyson and Eva have also bonded over their mutual love of cats. Their apartment is located just a few yards from a wooded area where they sometimes find feral cats. They also sometimes come across cats that are searching for scraps inside the apartment's dumpster. They take in the cats and care for them. They've kept several but have also found homes for some via the Internet. Yes, of course, I tell them the dangers of caring for feral cats (you should know me by now), but one thing about Greyson that hasn't changed a bit is his resistance to any and all advice from his mother. Eva has already contracted Lyme disease, which, of course, was on my list of Top Ten Reasons Why You Shouldn't Adopt Feral Cats. They both deny she contracted it from a cat, but clearly, she contracted it from a cat.

This may not be the happily-ever-after you were envisioning for Greyson, but this is the happiest he (and Eva) has ever been. They want to get married, but that would result in less government assistance for them, so they just wear inexpensive rings they purchased online and call each other husband and wife. I still periodically remind them not to procreate. Eva insists that she hates children and would never have them, and I love that about her. And fortunately, sex requires exuding energy, which goes against Greyson's sedentary beliefs. *Hallelujah, Magical Mattress God!*

This may not be the happily-ever-after you were anticipating for me, but I relish the days when Greyson and I have beautiful, intelligible conversations. I just wish they were the norm instead of the exception. (He's typically half-asleep or not very conversational.) Nothing else in the world makes me so happy and so sad at the same time than our nice conversations, which offer me flickers of what life would be like if I had a "normal" adult son.

I am, however, extremely happy to report that since Greyson is now seeing doctors regularly, taking a precise formula of prescription medications (that took years for Eva to perfect), and no longer having regular SAF episodes, our relationship has been mended, and I'm finally no longer afraid of him. And no longer feeling afraid of Greyson has clarified, for me, the ultimate goal of my book—to provide a stable home for him and Eva in the same city as me so I can visit and care for them.

Now, more than ever, I believe God works in mysterious ways. Years ago, I stopped praying for what I wanted God to do with Greyson. *Please Lord, heal Greyson's brain. Please Lord, keep Greyson off the streets. Please Lord, send Greyson to a facility where he'll receive useful help.* But never in a bazillion years would I have thought to pray, *Lord, please send Greyson a girl with a lifetime of experience with schizophrenia and extensive knowledge of prescription drugs. And if you wouldn't mind, it'd be great if she can live with Greyson, schedule his regular doctors' visits, escort him to every appointment, and ensure that he takes his meds daily. And Lord, while you're at it, can she make time to document his mood and behavioral changes and log the side effects he has to each medicine so the doctors can find an effective combination? And while I'm dreaming Lord, can she love him and want to be with him for the rest of his life? And on a side note Lord, it'd really help me out if you could pulverize her desire to reproduce. Got all that? Cool. Thanks, Lord.*

There's not a lot I'm sure about in life, but I do know that God helped Greyson find Eva—the only person on the planet who could help him—so there must be a purpose: a purpose for Greyson's life, for Eva's life, for my life. I won't pretend to know what our purpose is, but I do trust in Him.

Thank you for reading our story.

ACKNOWLEDGMENTS

My dear friend "Anna"—thank you for being the greatest friend I've ever had. You taught me to be kind, to dream big, and to always have dessert. I hope our story helps others, and I pray my delivery makes you proud.

Tiffany and Traci, thank you for donating your time with genuine love and care for my story. Your intuition and encouragement pushed me to dig deeper.

Thank you to my exceptional editor, Jennifer Huston. You are brilliant and insightful, but most importantly, you were an invaluable source of inspiration and support.

ABOUT THE AUTHOR

Claire Josephine has more than twenty-two years in the field of education. She lives with her children Violet and Rockwell and her two dogs. She is relocating to be closer to Greyson. *The Sad Son* is her first book.

Will Claire write again? Possibly. Follow her on social media to find out.

facebook.com/clairebjosephine
twitter.com/thesadsonauthor
instagram.com/clairebjosephine

Made in the USA
Las Vegas, NV
01 February 2021

16844337R00187